Healing Our ADHD Children

AN 8-WEEK PROGRAM FOR MOMS BY A MOM

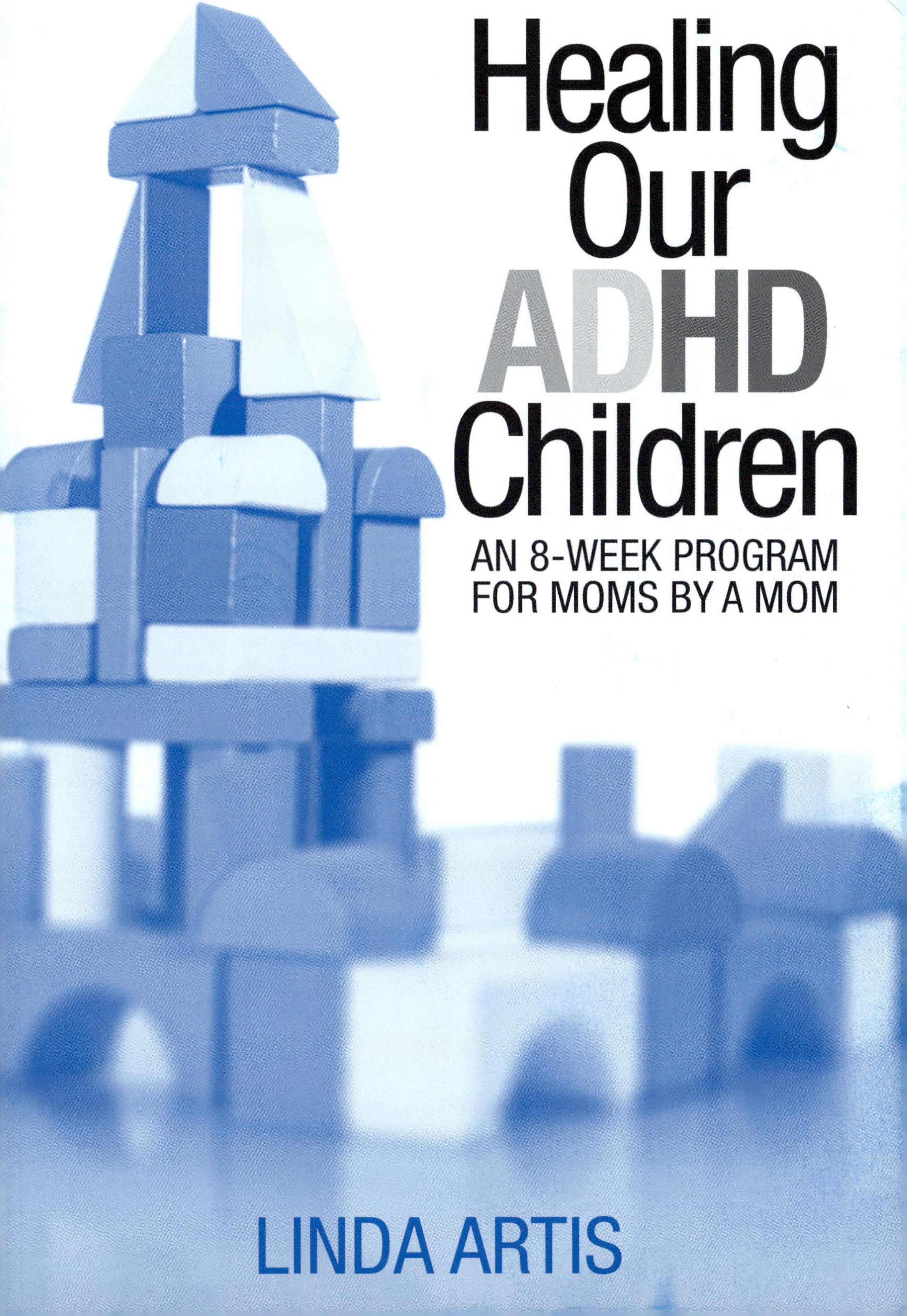

LINDA ARTIS

Healing Our ADHD Children:
An 8-Week Program for Moms by a Mom
By Linda Artis

Published by SPARK Publications

Design and production by SPARK Publications,
SPARKpublications.com

Printing History:
Edition One, May 2017, ISBN: 978-1-943070-22-0

Library of Congress Control Number: 2017937454

HEA032000 Alternative Therapies
HEA046000 Children's Health
HEA009000 Healing

Table of Contents

PART THREE: Interventions

Foreword & Disclaimer

For years I have been passionate about helping Moms with elementary school children. I am a Mom with a daughter and son who have been through many "diagnosis" in the past 10 years.

I have written this book to educate families and specifically Moms, on natural ways to eliminate the symptoms of attention deficit/hyperactivity disorder (ADHD), attention deficit disorder (ADD), oppositional defiant disorder (ODD), Asperger's syndrome, reactive attachment disorder (RAD), and dozens of other lesser-known diagnoses. I am not a doctor and do not have a medical degree. What I do have is common sense and a strong drive to find answers when the medical establishment fails us.

I know there are hundreds of ADHD books available. When I was contemplating writing this book, I went to Amazon and skimmed the first 250 books written on ADHD. Many were written by physicians, a handful were written by a parent, but I didn't find one that was written by a mom with an eight-week, building-block approach to eliminating your child's symptoms. This book is just that.

I have divided the book into an introduction and three unique sections. The introduction is the story of how our family adopted a son from Russia. I think you will enjoy reading it, and it will give you some context when you get to the section on discipline. However, the introduction, as well as each of the sections, stands alone and can be read in any order.

The first section is a culmination of years of experimentation related to toxin removal and supplementation and offers a special kid's elimination diet to determine food sensitivities. This is broken down into an eight-week program that is easy to follow. I believe that years from now doctors and scientists alike will discover that exposure to certain foods and certain toxins, which will be different for each child, is the number one cause of childhood illness. Eliminating these from your child's world will eliminate the ADHD or substantially lessen the symptoms.

The second section is on routines and discipline. Our children are different. Standard discipline techniques, such as timeouts, very seldom work for our children. This is a step-by-step approach to help our children learn how to function in our society and in our homes. I give many specific examples related to common situations we all find ourselves in on a regular basis.

The third section is a compilation of the most prevalent interventions that are available today for ADHD and the other diagnoses listed above. Some of these interventions eliminated symptoms, while others offered no improvement at all. Some are well publicized, but I have had limited exposure to them. When I have not personally tried an intervention, I have summarized the basic marketing material available to provide a general idea of what the intervention does and how it accomplishes the claimed results.

Throughout the book, I make suggestions or list products or ingredients by brand name. These are simply my preferences and are not paid endorsements.

Research and ADHD interventions are constantly changing. For my most current ADHD information and recent posts, visit my website at LindaArtis.com.

INTRODUCTION

To Russia and Back

They were dead. Not just one, but both of them. How could this have happened again? They were alive. They were growing. They were thriving! As the nurse continued to probe my belly, it was clear that there was no movement, no heartbeats—just silence. The joy of showing my 85-year-old mother what a fetus at three-months-old looks like and hearing the quiet but steady heartbeats melted into a despair that was almost too much to bear. I had been here before, but not this late in a pregnancy. Three months seemed to be some kind of bridge to life. If you make it over the three-month bridge, the chance that a baby will live and thrive increases exponentially. I thought I had made it, but I was wrong. There was nothing to do now but go through the long, drawn-out process of aborting the twins and bleeding. I think bleeding for many weeks must be a process to allow an expectant mom to grieve, but it seemed more of a constant reminder of my failure to get pregnant once again. Even after the bleeding finally stopped, there was an emotional bleeding process that would go on for months.

I reluctantly undertook the grieving process. My husband quickly moved on, seemingly unscarred by this blow to our hopes and dreams.

Thanks to the modern technology of in vitro fertilization (IVF), I already had a beautiful baby girl. She had just turned two years old and had been waiting patiently for siblings to arrive. The daily shots and constant blood draws were grueling, but somehow seemed worth every bit of it when that beautiful child was born. IVF was traumatic, painful and expensive, but we were willing to try again, for the chance at a second bundle of joy, or in this case a bonus of twins. It would not happen on that day or ever again for us. At some point the pain of constantly trying to biologically add to our current family had to end, and that was the day.

Far away, in a town called Pskov, Russia, a mother had a very different experience, and a baby was born in the springtime as the flowers bloomed and the trees pushed out their first new leaves. He was a healthy, eight-pound baby named Alexander. This baby didn't have a mother who would love and care for him. He did not have a mother who would feed him, bath him, wash away his tears, or laugh at the silly things he did. Instead, his mother was poor and scared, and one night, five days after Alexander was born, she quietly slipped away into the night and left her baby in the hands of the hospital staff. Being all too familiar with the plight the baby was in, they struggled to keep him alive on a limited budget until they could find someone to take care of him. Three months later he was moved to his second home in an orphanage, just a few miles away with more than a hundred children as roommates.

He lived as peacefully as possible in the orphanage until he was six months old, drinking bottles of formula as often as they were provided and waiting for a touch or a smile from one of the caregivers to come his way. Cribs were crammed together in a large room with barely enough space to walk between them. Babies cried constantly, and caregivers did their best given a terribly overcrowded situation. The room was clean, but it was hot and smelled of dirty diapers and sour milk. This small, fragile child eked out a pitiful existence day-by-day in his crib. Waiting.

Formula is expensive, and in an orphange on a limited budget, children are weaned off of a bottle and onto a substance called gruel as quickly as possible. This happened as Alexander turned seven months old. Alexander didn't like the gruel. He couldn't eat the gruel, and he threw up every time he was forced to eat it. His caregivers became increasingly frustrated as they barely had time to make the rounds to feed each child, without the additional worry of an increasingly thin, pale baby who could not eat the standard fare offered him. As Alexander continued to throw up, he became thinner, had a sickly tint to his skin, and lay in his crib and cried non-stop due to severe hunger pains. A decision was made to send him back to the hospital to try to save him from certain starvation.

On a cold, overcast winter day in February, Alexander was transported back to the hospital in a desperate attempt to save his life. People in scary white jackets came in and out of his room. They poked him with needles; they pushed on his stomach and stuck things down his throat. Occasionally, one of the white-jacket people would come and bring him some of the life-saving formula that he had thrived on the first six months of his existence. More pink started to creep into Alexander's cheeks, and he began feeling better. He gained a pound or two on the formula that was now his only nutritional source. Although the availability of formula was very limited, he was fed enough that his health continued to improve, and the hospital once again looked to the orphanage to take this baby and provide him with a stable environment to grow.

A First Meeting

There are a very limited number of ways to procure a family. One is obviously to have it yourself. Another is to adopt. Our attention turned toward the tedious process of adopting the remainder of our family. All my life I had dreamed of having three children, but at that point, I would have felt blessed to have two. Without the constraints of a pregnancy and X and Y chromosomes, we could now decide the gender of our second child. It would be a boy. Our daughter was growing quickly, and we wanted children as close together as possible in age. The adoption process in the United States seemed to be a crapshoot. We could put together a biography of ourselves, try to sell "us" to a potential mother to be, but would someone choose us over the hundreds or thousands of other couples wanting a baby? And what was the likelihood of that happening quickly? We wanted a process with a more definite outcome, so we turned to Russia. We were told that Russia had lots of boys that needed to be adopted and that we were almost guaranteed a baby boy within six months. The paperwork was daunting, so we hired a firm to fill out pages and pages for us. Five hectic months later in December, right before Christmas, we were boarding a plane for the 20-hour flight to St. Petersburg, Russia, to meet the baby boy that would soon complete our family.

Russia can be a daunting place to visit if you do not travel with a group or with a translator. We wandered around the streets, not understanding any of the strange words or letters that were all around us. Statues in small parks looked interesting, but we couldn't read the inscriptions. Restaurants looked good, but we had no idea what we were ordering. We managed to purchase a few souvenirs in a shop down the street and talked to a few college students who were excited to practice their English.

Our agency had arranged a transfer from the airport and then a second transfer to a region called Pskov a few days later. In between those times we were on our own. Lacking any idea of how or what to order in a restaurant, we found a small grocery market not far from our hotel where we recognized a few of the foods. We purchased cheese, crackers, chocolate, and beer, which sufficed for dinner. As we awoke the next morning ready for breakfast, but with no transportation, it was almost comical to grab our leftovers from the night before and feast on chocolate and cheese and wash it down with a beer. We were ready to face another day.

We were advised by our agency to exchange some money before we left for Russia. In addition, we were to bring $2,000 in American dollars in small bills for this first trip. Explicit instructions were given on who to pay and how much to pay. It was a mystery where the money went and who slipped money into whose pockets to make this whole process happen, although as far as we knew, it was legal. The driver showed up to transport us to our next destination. It was a four-hour ride to Pskov, and it would be a compliment to call the driver reckless. He drove up on curbs, around other cars, barely squeezing in between others, and the stoplights were clearly just suggestions. At times, all I could do was close my eyes and pray. Arriving at our destination, we slipped the driver $200 in crisp American bills and walked into the next hotel.

The hotel was set up for Americans who came in for adoptions, so registration and finding our room was easy. The hotel restaurant had pictures of the food, which made ordering somewhat easier. Thankfully there were a handful of other Americans there at the time. Although it was nice to talk to someone from our country, they were just as clueless as we were and couldn't offer any suggestions on places to eat or places to visit. We were confined to wandering around within a block or two of the hotel and eating our next six meals in the same hotel restaurant. The hour finally came for us to visit our soon-to-be son in the orphanage.

The orphanage was old and very rundown. It sat on a hill with a fenced-in area out back, but we were told that the children were never allowed to go outside because they could get sick. The orphanage was poorly lit, stifling hot, and smelled like the gruel fed to the older children. My stomach churned, but I managed to walk resolutely into the building and take a seat in the very small waiting room, anticipating meeting our child for the first time. We knew we would not be able to take this child home for almost two more months while Russian officials processed our paperwork. I braced for the emotional impact of meeting a baby I hoped would be mine; but nothing was guaranteed.

His name was Alexander. I could barely see his face when they brought him in. He was wrapped in blankets with a warm cap on his head. The room was even hotter than the rest of the building, and the child must have been roasting inside his blankets, but we were told not to take them off or he could get sick from a draft. We each held him, with a very surprising lack of emotion. This was just a child. He was not ours. I was sad that I couldn't make myself feel any attachment to the seven-month-old baby boy snuggled in my arms. I wondered if my husband felt the same way. It seemed more of a business transaction at this point. He would need to see a doctor to be sure he was healthy. He needed to be evaluated for fetal alcohol syndrome, which luckily he did not have. We had to approve of him and sign lots of paperwork so he could be our son. In a few hours we were back in our hotel room and two days later we were back in the United States, living the same life we lived before, hopeful that we could travel back in January to pick up our baby boy to complete our family.

The new year brought new regulations from the Russian government. A teenager who was adopted from Russia many years ago and brought to the United States had been murdered. The details never emerged through the media as to what happened, but Russians were mad that one of theirs had been mistreated. There was political pressure to stop Americans from adopting from Russia. Instead of stopping the whole process, the government put more paperwork in place and delayed the process. The new laws stated that Russians were the only ones allowed to adopt Russian children until they turned one. At that point, the child would be available for adoption by families from other countries.

Our agency completed all the new paperwork, but we couldn't travel until Alexander was one year old, which was five long months away. There was no correspondence, no pictures, no word on how he was doing. May rolled around, and we found ourselves back on a plane to St. Petersburg with a sense of excitement, but also one of caution. We completed this trip once. We could complete it again. The routine was more familiar the second time. We traveled from the U.S. to St. Petersburg and from St. Petersburg to Pskov with the same hair-raising car ride to the hotel. As we met our translator at the hotel there were new demands. Bring the orphanage diapers. Bring formula. Bring toys. Bring blankets and hats. The driver took us to a store to procure these. We did as we were told. We brought all the items we purchased to the orphanage and were allowed a short visit with Alexander.

Parents have to appear in front of a Russian judge and others at the courthouse to be approved in order to adopt a child. This was the last "test" we had to pass, and we were nervous and apprehensive. We got into the car for the 15-minute ride to the courthouse and were handed unexpected paperwork that we had not yet seen. As we read the medical page handed to us, we could only make out that Alexander was somehow sick. He had looked pale at the orphanage, but was so tightly swaddled in blankets and a hat that we hadn't seen the signs of starvation or sickness. He was a year old and weighed only 12 pounds. Unknown to us until that minute, he had been in the hospital for months, and the best we could make out from the paperwork we were quickly trying to decipher was a diagnosis of reflux because nothing else could be found. The translator wanted to know if we still wanted to adopt the child. How could we possibly process this whole new health situation in just 10 minutes? We had spent thousands of dollars and traveled twice to Russia. Our family was invested in the outcome. How could we leave without the child even if he was terribly sick? The situation was not what we signed up for. We felt like we had been tricked into taking a child that had major health issues.

We left the Russian courtroom holding Alexander, a one-year-old baby boy who had become ours—ours to care for and comfort, ours to feed (if that was even possible based on his medical diagnosis), ours to raise for the next 17 years and ours as part of our family forever. There was a knot in my stomach and an empty place in my heart that over time would have to fill up with love for this new child.

The trip back from Russia was a hard one. We spent one last night in the hotel in Pskov. The hotel management didn't have any cribs, so they put a cot in our room for our new child. We didn't get much sleep that night. The next evening we boarded an overnight train for Moscow. We had our own sleeper car, but it was stifling hot. When we opened the door, which was our only way to get fresh air, our new baby continued to crawl out the door and around the train. No sleep that night. We finally fell asleep in the wee hours of the morning but were awakened abruptly as shouts came through the train to be sure everyone had debarked. It was the end of the line, and everyone was off the train except us! We frantically grabbed our stuff, grabbed our baby, and hustled off the train. Russians glared at us because in our haste we had forgotten to put Alexander's hat on his head, which apparently proved what horrible parents we had just become.

We rested in Moscow for a couple of days and with our new baby in tow, we were able to enjoy this fabulous city and some of its many architectural wonders. Twenty hours of flights through multiple different airports brought us safely back to the United States and the start of a tumultuous life with our second child.

Routines and Adjustments

Being back in the United States presented its own set of challenges. My husband and I were now Alexander's fourth caretakers in a year. My husband had a full-time job, and I had a part-time job and would eventually have to go back to work. In three months, Alexander would be sent to daycare with a new routine to get used to, new people to learn to love, and new foods to eat. Not wanting the situation to unfold in that way, we reasoned that if he spent a few hours a day in his future daycare environment, we might spare him the trauma of getting used to a fourth caretaker, which was us and then moving to a fifth caretaker, which was the daycare.

We immediately enrolled him in daycare, and to our astonishment, he thrived. There were other children, which was similar to the orphanage. There were six cribs lined up next to each other, which was at least a little like the orphanage, and there were caretakers. Although for us it was a stretch to compare any part of this new daycare to the atrocities of the orphanage, in some small way it must have reminded him of it and given him some sense of belonging, or at least a sense of familiarity. He was happy, content, and thriving in this new environment.

Unfortunately, home life was just the opposite. Every day I would wake up tired and irritable from intermittent sleep. I woke up twice each night to feed him a bottle of formula, just like a newborn. In the morning he would wake up screaming for another bottle. Alex, which is what we now called him, had intense hunger pains, but the brutal awakening and the rush to get him a bottle was only the first hurdle of the day. As the day progressed, I would sit on the floor in the playroom trying to engage him in an activity. The attention span of all babies is short, but after a brief period of time to inspect the toy I had to offer, Alex would crawl through a short hallway and into the kitchen. He would sit and scream for food. He had eaten breakfast only an hour before, so I would bring him back to the playroom and offer up another toy, once again with the same results. Exhausted after many iterations of this same behavior, I would give in and sit on the kitchen floor feeding him one Cheerio at a time for hours until lunchtime rolled around. Taking Alex to the park elicited the same response. All the other kids were on the slide or swings, jumping, running, playing. Alex was in his stroller as I handed him one Cheerio at a time to fill his starved little body. I always wondered if I was losing the battle. I could only imagine that his body burned that Cheerio faster than he could mush it up in his mouth and get it down to his stomach. It was heart-wrenching to watch this day after day.

Alex had sensory issues and would throw up every time he ate anything lumpy, except for Cheerios. Even applesauce was too lumpy for him. Baby food, formula, and a constant supply of Cheerios started to slowly bring some color back to his cute face, but he was still nothing but skin and bones underneath his clothes. We were frustrated with this child who threw up daily for unknown reasons and was seldom happy at home. The pediatrician was baffled, but since he was eating, we kept doing the same thing and hoped he would outgrow it. He was gaining some weight, building some muscle, and did not look as sickly as when he had arrived in America.

One night I had spent the normal hour it took to feed Alex his dinner. This took an exceeding amount of patience because he ate slowly and was extremely messy. It was closer to the task of feeding a six month old, only he ate twice as much. Alex was unable to feed himself because every Cheerio and every spoonful of food would find its way quickly to the floor. He refused to put even a spoonful into his mouth. I could only think that in the orphanage, the more things he dropped on the floor the better the chances of having a caregiver come over to pick up something and give him a pat on the back or a kind word. Even if he was constantly starved, he craved the attention more than the food. I took him down from the high chair and placed him in his favorite spot in the middle of the kitchen floor. I walked over to the sink to put away the spoon and containers. Then I heard a slight gagging sound, and when I turned around, I almost cried. There was Alex in the middle of the floor. All the baby food I had so painstakingly fed him was in pools all around him and all over his body. It was as if I had set a baby in the middle of the floor and poured a couple of jars of baby food on and around him. It made me briefly wonder if the best thing to do wouldn't be to get the spoon and just start putting it back in his mouth. I promise I didn't!

Three months later we were visiting the neighborhood park with some friends. It was lunchtime, so my friend suggested we order a pizza for park delivery. I had a supply of Cheerios for Alex, so this sounded like a great idea for the rest of us. The warm pizza arrived, and it smelled heavenly with hot gooey cheese and pepperoni on top. One of the children gave Alex a piece, and before I realized it, he had eaten half of it. I ran for the wipes and towels to clean up the impending mess, but nothing happened. Alex happily ate an entire piece of pizza and never threw up food again! I could only shake my head at this sudden, bizarre change of eating habits.

A Challenging Child

Alex turned two years old in late spring when it seemed everyone in our family should be peaceful and happy. Alex should have been steadily adjusting to his new life, but he wasn't. He had adjusted beautifully to the daycare environment, but home life was a constant struggle. Other than throwing up about once a week because he ate too much and didn't realize it, his food issues had disappeared. He had more than doubled his weight and was likely headed for basketball player status as he was in the 90th percentile for height at his two-year annual physical.

Although Alex's physical needs were being met, his emotional needs were the bigger issue. He was fussy all the time, and I compared him to a newborn with colic. It was hard to bond with him due to the constant tears and fits of rage. We reasoned that when he had caught up on his weight and wasn't so hungry, most of this might disappear on its own. We prayed for him to start talking once he turned two, so he could tell us what he needed. It was heart-wrenching to feel more like his babysitter than his mother. The case worker would come in every so often, look at Alex, tell us he was bonding just fine, write some things on her sheet of paper, and leave. We hoped we were doing the right thing. We were giving him a home with as much love as we could muster for this bundle of almost constant fussiness.

As we thought things were starting to settle down a bit, Alex was almost three years old when he hit his full blown terrible twos. My daughter had experienced this childhood phenomena a few years back, so I thought I knew what to expect. She had thrown her share of tantrums, but like most children, she quickly realized that tantrums only produced a mother that walked away and a dessert or a toy that was even more unattainable after the fury she had unleashed. Her tantrum stage was short lived, but cropped up occasionally, just in case Mom changed her mind.

Alex was an entirely different child. With emotional trauma in his past, his terrible twos took on a new meaning. He would find something minor about which to complain and then have a temper tantrum that would last up to an hour in length. I didn't think that was physically possible, but he wailed and cried and screamed for a long, long time. It was like a battle of wills. I wouldn't give in and give him what he wanted, and he wouldn't stop screaming. Even though he never got what he wanted and didn't get any attention during these episodes, in some way I think these tantrums must have soothed him or given him something he needed. He could have five or six tantrums a day because he picked the arguments. In the car, he would tell me to go left when he knew his daycare was to the right. Since I didn't do what he asked, he would scream and wail the rest of the way to daycare each morning. I would make him a dinner that I knew he liked, but he would complain that the corn was too hot and would demand that I make him a different meal. When I refused to give in, he would scream and wail and ultimately not get any dinner at all.

Alex continued this behavior for years. We tried many interventions. We started with the Pediatrician, and at the age of six, Alex was diagnosed with ADHD. He couldn't sit still, he talked and asked questions which constantly interrupted the teacher and he didn't get social cues that he should be learning at this age. By first grade, the teacher pulled his desk away from everyone else and sat him next to her desk facing her. He was angry and embarrassed. In second and third grade we worked through food sensitivity testing, behavior modification with a Psychologist and various medications.

As we went through different interventions, we would take two steps forward and one step backward. Sometimes it seemed like we would take two steps backward and one step forward. We were, however, making progress, and Alex's behavior continued to improve. Today, he is very different than the child who would scream in anger many times a day. Although Alex can still be stubborn and controlling, those traits have been tempered with a new sense of responsibility, perseverance, determination, and love.

You will read stories about Alex throughout this book, as well as about my daughter, whom I will introduce later. I will give you step-by-step strategies and suggestions on what to try with a child not growing up "by the book". You may not currently have a diagnosis for your child, but suspect that something is wrong. Your child may already have a diagnosis of attention deficit/hyperactivity disorder (ADHD), oppositional defiant disorder (ODD) or Asperger's. Many adopted children not only have ODD and ADHD, but also have a condition called Reactive Attachment Disorder (RAD) which manifests itself mainly as an insatiable need to control everything around them. Many years after I started on this journey and Alex had been diagnosed with ADHD, Alex was re-diagnosed with RAD.

In a medical world that tries to treat every child the same, the glaring fact remains that every child is different and modern medicine is not setup to heal our children individually. Doctors are setup to eliminate as many symptoms as possible to help with day-to-day struggles and they do that by prescribing medications. This book is setup to heal and eliminate the symptoms of our ADHD, ADD, ODD, and RAD children forever. We want our kids to live healthy, productive lives and, if at all possible, live those lives without medications and side effects that will hinder their well-being either now or in the future.

I pray that this book and some of the things that I have learned over many years can help moms to short-cut the process. There are so many avenues down which you can turn. I have turned down many of them, sometimes successfully and sometimes not so successfully. It is also probable that every mom will get different results than I got with my children and also different results than every other mom. Every child that suffers from ADHD, ADD, ODD, Asperger's, RAD, and others manifests symptoms in slightly different ways. The same answer is not right for every child.

Every mom and child will emerge from these eight-week programs with different results. One child might show food sensitivities to gluten, red dye 40 and have a deficiency of Magnesium and Vitamin D. Another child might have food sensitivities to corn, eggs and sugar and have a bad reaction to hand sanitizers. The possibilities are endless. That is the nature of this epidemic and why a building-block approach to these childhood epidemics is so important. Once you know how your child reacts to toxins and different foods, then eliminating the offending substances can produce a child free of the symptoms causing so much frustration in your family today.

PART ONE:

Food Sensitivities

CHAPTER 1

Diagnosing ADHD and Other Disorders

If you are reading this book, you likely have a good idea that your child is struggling more than other children. If you are looking for a diagnosis, there are lists of questions in many ADHD books to help. In addition, your pediatrician will also have a set of questions to be answered by you and your child's teachers in order to establish a diagnosis. The psychiatrist my husband and I visited for our son let us know that the reason it is so important to get an accurate diagnosis is so that we can then seek the proper treatment for our son. As I began wading through the possible treatments for ADHD, it occurred to me how ambiguous that statement was. "Proper treatment" is defined differently based on which type of professional you decide to visit.

Pediatricians try to help by prescribing medications based on their medical knowledge. Few pediatricians have knowledge of food sensitivities, discipline techniques, school situations, and other factors that can substantially alter or even eliminate ADHD behavior. Instead, they do the best they can to address the symptoms, by doing the only thing they are trained to do. They prescribe medications, usually stimulants such as Focalin, Adderall or Ritalin, that mask ADHD and help families to live with the disorder on a permanent basis. I am not saying this is a bad approach, only that this is just one of many different approaches. Your pediatrician may suggest that this is the only viable treatment for ADHD, in which case I would say your doctor is incorrect. If he is not willing to consider other options, a different pediatrician might be a good decision.

Consider someone who is not feeling well and doesn't know where to turn. Let's say they have chronic shoulder pain, but it could be a symptom related to hundreds of different conditions or injuries. If this person visits a medical doctor, that doctor will likely prescribe drugs, such as steroids. If this person visits a chiropractor, they will get back and neck adjustments. If they visit a sports medicine doctor, they will be sent for physical therapy. If they visit a psychologist, they will go to sessions to help reduce their anxiety and stress, which could be the cause of the underlying pain. None of these approaches are wrong. Each doctor believes they have the cure for your symptoms, but few of them will acknowledge that there may be other ways to cure your pain. Can you see how the same scenario plays out when your child receives an ADHD diagnosis?

My daughter was diagnosed with ADD at the end of third grade. I started with the pediatrician, moved to combing the Internet for answers, tried vitamin and mineral supplementation and something called Bender Breakthrough, which was a regiment of crawling exercises, and then dabbled in food elimination. Because none of this helped much, I moved to medications for a couple of years. From there I moved her to a much smaller school that could work with her distractibility and auditory processing issues and discontinued the medication. I handled the distractibility at home mostly through the discipline interventions in part two of this book. Sometimes she is in the middle of doing one thing and all of a sudden loses focus and moves on to something else. Our word for that is "squirrel" just as a dog will be minding his own business, but if he sees a squirrel, his focus changes in a nanosecond! If I am around when this happens, I say "squirrel" and she immediately understands what she just did and can go back to her previous task. We always laugh!

In high school, she needed to go back to the medication only for semester exams, which were three to five hours in length. To handle one particularly boring morning class, she resorted to a cup of coffee each morning, which did the same thing as the stimulant drugs but wasn't time released, so it wore off more quickly. Nevertheless it got her through a tough biology class that was predominantly a lecture.

If I had known when she was in elementary school about an eight-week program such as the one you are about to read in this book, I would have had a different outcome today. Unfortunately, once kids get to middle school and high school it is much more difficult to get through an elimination diet. There are sleep overs and get togethers with peer pressure to eat whatever is there. They have likely either figured out how to live with their limitations or are on medication and have figured out how to live with the side effects. It is much easier to motivate younger children when it comes to an elimination diet. They are still at the age where they need your approval and want to please you and you can make it fun if you enlist their help.

If you read the Introduction in this book, you will already know a little bit about my son and the circumstances that brought him into my life. At an early age he was diagnosed with ADHD but had a much harder time than my daughter. The H (which stands for hyperactive) presented real problems. Without the H, a child can sometimes slip through the cracks and not be noticed. It is hard not to notice the hyperactivity of an ADHD child, and later that H might morph into additional diagnosis like ODD or Asperger's or any number of other less-well-known diagnoses. Many interventions that I tried for my son are listed in part three Interventions. These include interventions for ADHD as well as Reactive Attachment Disorder (RAD), which is a diagnosis he received later on in Elementary School.

It is our job as parents to determine how we want to handle our children's diagnoses. Do we want to treat the symptoms with medication, or do we want to try other interventions to help overcome the symptoms or even eliminate them? There will almost always be a building-block approach, depending on the situation. This might include putting a child on medication first, to help with the day-to-day struggles, while exploring other options. Another way to approach this is to explore other options first and go to medication as a last resort. There are no right or wrong answers—only what works best for each of our families trying to do the best we can for our children.

Interventions related to doctors will be covered later, but for now, if you feel you must work with a professional, I would highly recommend a functional doctor, a naturopathic doctor, or a homeopathic doctor. Functional doctors will do an initial screening and then recommend various testing. After an analysis of test results, certain supplements will be recommended, and foods will be added or eliminated from your child's diet. There will be a large upfront cost for these services, as the initial testing is expensive, but not as much of an ongoing cost. Naturopathic and homeopathic doctors work in a similar fashion but are not as expensive on the front end. They will typically determine what supplements or herbs to prescribe based on an extensive questionnaire, detailed discussions, or sometimes based on a practice called kinesiology, which relates to human movement and energy flow in the body. They might also try to determine food sensitivities through various testing and talk about how to remove chemicals from your household. If you would like to medicate your child to mask some of his or her symptoms, then a pediatrician is the appropriate doctor to consult. Later on if your child needs additional medications, there are doctors that specialize in multiple medications for childhood symptoms such as ODD and Asperger's.

This section will walk you through an eight-week program that will recommend vitamins and minerals most ADHD children are deficient in, focus on eliminating toxins and chemicals from your child's environment and will determine if your child has food sensitivities. Part two will address certain behaviors that still may not have improved after the first eight weeks due to bad habits that need to be corrected. Part three lists additional mainstream interventions and includes some commentary on each in case you are still looking for additional suggestions after completing the first two sections.

No matter which way you turn, it is important to face the fact that your child does indeed have a diagnosis that can't be ignored. Don't waste time hoping your child is just a little hyperactive or just a slow learner or just a rambunctious boy or girl. The testing most pediatricians do is easy and will quickly let you know what the initial diagnosis is. You can't fix anything until you acknowledge there is a problem!

When my daughter was in kindergarten, she didn't know all her letters or shapes. When she started first grade, she could barely read a book with one sentence on each page. By second grade, she was having trouble with her addition and was falling behind in general. Something happened in second grade that changed my perspective. Her teacher asked for parent volunteers to come in for an hour during the children's independent work time each day. I volunteered every Friday. When I arrived at school, I would check off their reading from the night before, hang things on the wall, or sometimes help a small group with their reading. Most importantly, I was able to watch my child while I was doing these other things. What an eye opener! Although I was aware that she couldn't sit still at the dinner table and her homework was almost impossible to complete each night, watching her in school and comparing her to 24 other children was something for which I was not prepared. She changed positions in her seat at least every 30 seconds. She looked around. She played with her pencil. She did everything except listen to the teacher. It was like her "On" button was stuck. All the other children could turn their buttons off long enough to listen to the teacher and the instructions before they got busy with another assignment. My child did not seem to have an "Off" button. After the instructions were given, she looked around with no idea what to do. If I had known better at the time, I would have diagnosed her on the spot with ADD or maybe ADHD. It was almost two years later when I finally took her to the pediatrician and received an official ADD diagnosis.

When my son started first grade, the diagnosis was easy. I volunteered to help with a party. In less than an hour in the classroom, I could pick out three children that I was sure had ADHD and one that was on the edge. Alex definitely had ADHD. I had him evaluated by the pediatrician, filled out all the questionnaires and confirmed the diagnosis.

Unfortunately, teachers are not allowed to bring up the subject or make a diagnosis, for fear of not following the rules or labeling students. You can try to ask the teacher, "Do you think my child has ADHD? I want an honest opinion." This is really scary to ask, and there are many teachers who will refuse to answer the question, but it is worth a try. When I suspected my daughter had ADD, I didn't want to ask. What if, by asking, I made this diagnosis real? If I didn't ask, maybe it would just go away, and I wouldn't have to label my child with something I didn't know anything about. Please don't stick your head in the sand like I did and hope it goes away. I wasted two valuable years of my child's life doing this, and I wish I could get those two years back. I would have saved my child a lot of heartache and painful times if I had tackled this thing immediately instead wishing it would resolve itself.

Genetics or Toxins

Autism, ADD, ADHD, and ODD are part of our children's world, and Alzheimer's, multiple sclerosis, psoriasis, lupus, and hundreds of new autoimmune diseases are part of our adult world. There are disagreements, even within the medical community as to whether these disorders are genetic or caused by other unknown factors. If we say they are genetic, as many physicians believe, then it is much easier to prescribe medications since genetic implies there is nothing else we can do to eliminate the symptoms.

Let's use a common-sense approach and take a second look at this theory. If all of these relatively new diseases were genetic, why didn't we see the same symptoms in children and adults years ago? The Centers for Disease Control and Prevention (CDC) puts the number of children between ages four and 17 who have ADHD at 11 percent or roughly 6.4 million children. If this was a genetic disease, how did we go from less than 1 percent to 11 percent in less than 100 years? The study of genetics would tell you that it is rare, if not impossible, for a genetic mutation to propagate through the human population that dramatically in such a short period of time. It is also ridiculous to say that all of these disorders existed 100 years ago, but we just didn't know what to call them. Some doctors will say that there is an extreme ADHD over-diagnosis, but even if you believe that, there are simply too many kids today with ADHD and other secondary diagnoses to think that this same number of kids was misdiagnosed a hundred years ago or that a substantial number of these kids are misdiagnosed today. The chart below points out that even in the past 18 years, combining both girls and boys, ADHD has increased from 5.5 percent to almost 9 percent of children ages three to 17, which represents over 2 million additional diagnoses.

Figure 1

Percentage of Children Ages 3-17 with Attention Deficit-Hyperactivity Disorder (ADHD), by Gender, 1997-2013

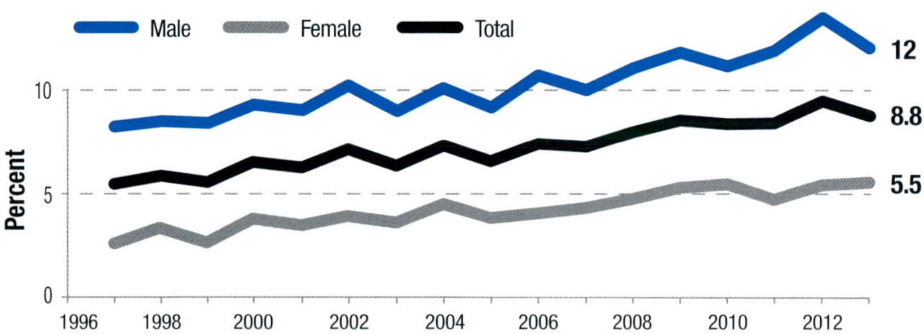

Source: Original analysis by Child Trends of National Health Interview Survey data 1997-2013.

Saying that our kid's ADHD is caused by their genetic make-up and by extension, there is nothing to be done except medicate them is irresponsible. We had a similar genetic make-up 100 years ago, but the difference is that we were not exposed to thousands of chemicals in our houses, our water, our air and our food. Julie Buckley in her book *Healing Our Autistic*

Children describes autism as "the neurological and biological expression of the impact of environmental toxins on genetically susceptible kids." I believe ADHD, ADD, ODD, and autoimmune diseases have the same definition. Some humans are genetically more susceptible to some substances than other substances. Just as some people have allergies to pollen, and some don't. That is genetic. Some people are highly allergic to peanuts, and some are not. That is genetic. I believe that most of our kids are sensitive—not allergic (I will explain this later)—to chemicals and additives in our current food supply. This manifests itself as ADHD. That is genetic. The point is that genetics didn't cause these problems. What caused the problems is that our environment has become riddled with thousands of toxins in our food, our water and our air, and the children and adults that are genetically predisposed to these toxins are getting sick. Children are getting autism, ADHD, ADD, ODD, and others. Adults are getting autoimmune diseases because the toxins in our environment are ruining our immune systems. That is genetic, but it does not mean that drugs are the answer. The answer lies in defining and eliminating the toxins to which we have sensitivies and thus reducing symptoms or completely eliminating the disease.

It is reasonable to think that ADHD, ODD, Asperger's, asthma, food allergies, learning disabilities, sensory processing disorders, and many others are all on the same spectrum. Reactions to more than 80,000 toxins in our world manifest differently in different children with different gene pools. The bottom line is that getting these toxins out of our day-to-day lives can dramatically alter our children's behavior.

As you will read later in this book, there are many different ways to moderate or even eliminate symptoms of ADHD. This section is on eliminating symptoms based on environmental and nutritional toxins. As our society continues to use an overwhelming array of toxins for everything from cleaning the floors to washing our clothes, we expose our children, with their undeveloped bodies and brains, to these toxins.

Then we continue to bombard their small, developing bodies by giving them foods to ingest that include dyes, preservatives, MSG, toxic chemicals used on GMO foods, and more. The unfortunate little bodies that happen to be more genetically susceptible to these toxins may develop any range of diseases.

Week 2 of the eight-week program in this section will walk you through eliminating as many toxins from your environment as possible.

Allergies and Food Sensitivities

I have used the term "food sensitivities" a number of times already, so I would like to talk about the difference between food sensitivities and food allergies before we jump into a food sensitivity elimination diet. A food allergy exists when a person's immune system has an unwanted reaction to a particular food. The body mistakes the food as harmful and calls on the bodies' defense system of antibodies to fight the invasion. The immune system immediately releases histamines, which cause the reaction we observe, such as hives, itchy eyes, welts, or a more severe reaction, such as trouble breathing or anaphylaxis. Food sensitivity or food intolerance is a digestive system response rather than an immune system response. This happens when a food is digested that irritates the stomach lining or intestinal tract, and the food cannot be properly digested.

The body responds quickly to an allergy, whereas a food sensitivity might take hours or even days to create a reaction. When a person has an allergy, even a small amount of a food can trigger a life-threatening reaction in severe cases. Many times people can tolerate small amounts of a food if they have a food sensitivity. They might feel exhausted, have stomach cramps, bloating, headaches, or other less apparent symptoms. The food sensitivity might affect the way a child behaves or it might affect his or her ability to pay attention or learn in a classroom. Since their brain is still growing, it might affect executive functioning or social learning or any number of other learned behaviors. There are some mainstream tests administered to determine childhood allergies. There are less effective blood tests available for food sensitivities, which I do not recommend (more in part three on this). In my experience, a food elimination diet is the best, least expensive and the most effective way to test for food sensitivities.

The Feingold Program

Before we get into toxin removal and the elimination diet, I would like to spend some time introducing the Feingold Program. The Feingold Association of the United States, a nonprofit that has been in existence since 1976, runs the program. The main Feingold diet eliminates dyes, artificial sweeteners, artificial flavors, and preservatives including BHA, BHT, and TBHQ (see glossary for definitions). There is also a special diet program for people sensitive to salicylates, which include some common fruits and vegetables (more on this later).

Most children's food studies conducted between 1976, when Feingold began and 1995 were related to sensitivity of children to dyes. Skeptics said that the studies' were inconclusive because outcomes were all over the board. Based on the chart below, we can see why this might be.

Challenge Studies *Results appear to be "all over the place"*

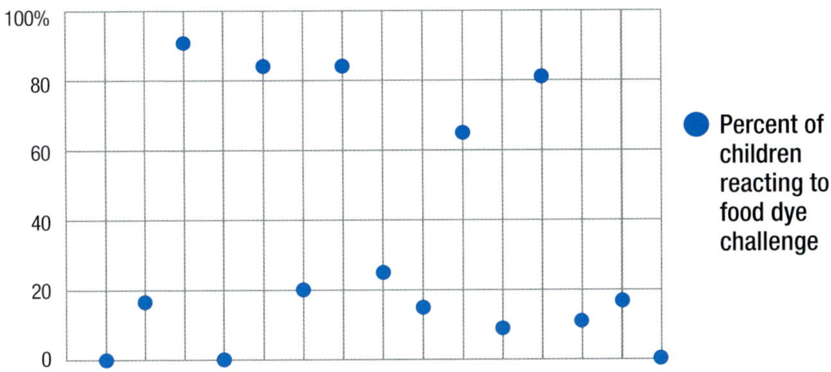

However, Feingold took these studies and rearranged them based on the amount of dyes given to the children during the study. As this next chart shows, when children ingest more than 50 mg of dyes per day, anywhere from 60% to 90% reacted with behavioral issues. When the dyes were removed from their diets, the children showed a substantial improvement in behavior, learning and general health.

Graphed against mg of dye used *It is a dose-response!!*

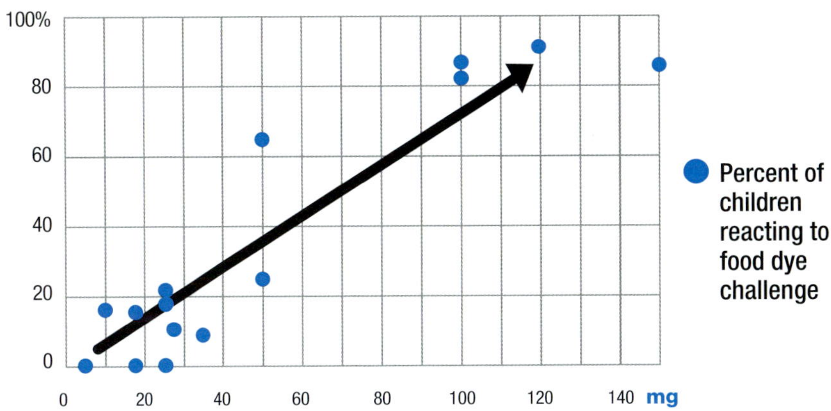

Most of our children can easily consume 100 mg to 300 mg of dyes per day. Giving your child one 16 ounce Kool-Aid Burst Cherry drink would result in them ingesting 104.6 mg of dyes and a 16 ounce Powerade Orange results in 44.2 mg being ingested according to a study published in Clinical Pediatrics in February 2014.

Since this time, there have been hundreds of studies conducted not only for sensitivity to dyes, but also for sensitivity to preservatives, salicylates, gluten, casein and other offenders. As of the writing of this book, Feingold has published 93 of these studies on their website for further review.

Unfortunately, this is not something your pediatrician is likely to tell you. The majority of pediatricians have become so entrenched with the pharmaceutical companies that they are most comfortable prescribing drugs for our children. The medical education they received probably had limited information on foods and chemicals and how those affect our bodies, so they are not comfortable with this subject. Most will simply provide a prescription to cover up ADHD symptoms. What we need to do is heal our children's ADHD symptoms, instead of masking them with medicine.

Although it is not a requirement, I highly recommend taking a look at the Feingold program and what it offers and consider joining the group. As I recommend different foods to eat, I will sometimes refer back to the Feingold Foodlist.

The Feingold Program produces an updated Foodlist on a yearly basis. A questionnaire is sent to food producers to verify the actual ingredients in each food that is recommended on the list. This is a very time-consuming process, as hundreds of brands are included in the inquiries. Our sketchy laws related to ingredient lists don't always include toxic ingredients, so it is necessary to vet out the chemicals that are harmful to highly sensitive children and adults. An example of this is the use of the ingredient called "Natural flavoring", which is included in thousands of different products. The Food and Drug Administration (FDA) allows "Natural flavoring" to be used in ingredient labels to include any ingredient that is not synthetic or manmade. Basically, it is not necessary for food producers to ever divulge their true ingredient lists. In my opinion, it is well worth the annual subscription fee to obtain a copy of this food list and to join the mailing list to receive their very informative newsletters.

Let's take a closer look at the offending chemicals that Feingold helps to identify and remove from our diets.

Food Dyes

Artificial food dyes are made from petroleum and have increased in use over the past 50 years by more than 500 percent. There have been numerous studies conducted in an effort to link these dyes to hyperactivity in children. Enough studies were performed that substantiated this link that the European Union in 2010 started requiring a label on all dyed foods that says "may have an adverse effect on activity and attention in children." Since this time, the majority of dyes have been eliminated from foods in Europe. Countries such as Norway, Finland, France, Austria, and the UK have banned dyes such as Red 40, Blue 1, and six others that food companies in the United States routinely use. The FDA, with increasing pressure from big food companies has chosen to look the other way and continues to allow food our children consume to be laced with these chemicals, despite the growing body of evidence that they can cause many ADHD and ODD symptoms.

Artificial Sweeteners

Studies continue to prove that artificial sweeteners such as sucralose (Splenda) and aspartame (Equal) cause a myriad of health issues and negative reactions can be compounded when ingested by children with developing brains and bodies. If your children are currently drinking or eating foods with these sweeteners, please remove them from their diets. Look for foods that contain cane sugar, which is substantially better than using these sweeteners. Contrary to standard marketing hype, there is no current evidence that suggests that children or adults lose weight or keep from gaining weight by eating foods containing artificial sweeteners. In fact, some new studies suggest that artificial sweeteners play havoc with our bodies' natural hunger signals and make us feel hungry when we are really not hungry. This can lead to overeating and weight gain.

Artificial Flavors and Natural Flavors

The difference between artificial and natural flavors is that natural flavors are created from anything that can be eaten such as fruits, vegetables, or animals. Artificial flavors are derived from anything that is typically considered inedible such as petroleum. A chemical such as vanillin, which is a cheap knockoff of natural vanilla, would be considered an artificial flavor. Fifteen years ago, vanillin was mostly made from waste produced by the sulfite pulping process for preparing wood pulp for the paper industry. Today, it is typically made from petrochemicals. In 2006, Japanese researcher Mayu Yamamoto won the 2007 Nobel Chemistry Prize for figuring out how to extract a substance from cow poop that tasted the same as vanillin. That would then be listed in our ingredient list as a "natural flavor" or "vanillin." Castoreum is another flavoring used for it's vanilla taste and would be considered a natural flavor. It is derived from castor sacs located under a beaver's tail, next to the anal glands. Yuck! I guess the point is that a consumer has no idea what natural or artificial flavoring really is, so we don't know whether our kids are sensitive to it or not. It is best to avoid all foods that have either of these two ingredients in the ingredient list located on food packaging.

Preservatives Including BHA, BHT and TBHQ

BHA and BHT are widely used in the food industry as preservatives. Their main job is to prevent oil in foods from oxidizing and becoming rancid. Enough animal studies have been performed that have caused the National Toxicology Program to conclude that BHA should be "reasonably anticipated to be a human carcinogen." Avoid these preservatives by reading ingredient labels carefully and staying away from processed foods.

Salicylates

The Feingold Program was the first group to bring the idea that people could be sensitive to salicylates into the food sensitivity discussion. It is postulated that certain fruits and vegetables include a chemical called salicylates that is naturally occurring but can cause a sensitivity in some children. Natural foods with high amounts of salicylates include:

Almonds	Coffee	Pickles
Apples	Cucumbers	Pineapple (Fresh)
Apricots	Currants	Plums
Aspirin	Dates	Prunes
Berries (all)	Grapes	Raisins
Bell Peppers	Oil of Wintergreen	Rose Hip
Cherries	Oranges	Tea
Cloves	Peaches	Zucchini

The elimination of these mostly wholesome foods has caused some backlash toward the Feingold Program over the years. Fewer children are sensitive to salicylates than to larger offending food groups, such as gluten and dairy. However, as new studies are conducted, certain salicylates are starting to show up as culprits in various autoimmune diseases, such as tomatoes, coffee, and almonds. It follows that these may also be culprits in our children's ADHD diagnoses.

Our kids typically have low levels of an enzyme called PST in the liver that is responsible for processing salicylates through the body. Salicylates can cause additional irritation for children with leaky gut syndrome, yeast overgrowth, or an overload of toxins from various other foods.

We will be removing salicylates for the elimination diet but will add back a few of these foods early in the diet, looking for any adverse reactions as we go. Look carefully at the foods above so that you don't accidentally feed your child any of these while working through the elimination diet.

Genetically Modified Foods (GMOs)

Although GMO foods are not currently included as a separate category in the Feingold Program, they have risen to the top of the list of controversial foods in our society. Today GMO foods include soy, corn, cotton, canola, sugar beets, alfalfa, papaya, yellow summer squash, and zucchini squash. In 2015, the FDA approved GMO salmon, GMO apples and GMO potatoes. A gene was inserted into apples and potatoes to keep them from turning brown after being cut open and sitting exposed for a period of time. In addition, GMO crops such as soy, corn, alfalfa, and cottonseed are used to feed the majority of our livestock.

So what exactly is a GMO food? In 1994, scientists introduced the first foods that were tolerant to chemical herbicides commonly used on farms. Herbicides such as RoundUp, which contains the poison called glyphosate, were produced and sold by Monsanto, a giant chemical company in the United States. Monsanto is the same company that has developed GMO crops. Scientists removed certain DNA from the seeds of the foods listed above, and inserted new DNA into genes that would keep the plants from dying when sprayed with chemicals such as RoundUp.

Unknown to scientists at the beginning of this GMO experiment, more and more weeds grew in the farmer's fields after using GMO seeds.

This meant that farmers had to use an increasing amount of chemicals to control the weeds. Just two years after introducing GMO crops, a study in Australia showed that seven to 11 times more weeds were growing due to GMO crops. This means that more chemicals need to be used to kill the extra weeds. According to a study by Environmental Sciences Europe (*Impacts of Genetically Engineered Crops on Pesticide Use in the US – The First Sixteen Years*), herbicide use has increased between 1996 and 2011 by 527 million pounds due to herbicide-resistant superweeds. The logical conclusion is that humans are now being exposed to this additional chemical usage created by GMO plants. There have been numerous studies linking these chemicals to kidney and liver damage, toxicity in the brain, cell malformations, and many others. It makes sense to think these same chemicals could be a major disruptor in our children's brains.

If this wasn't bad enough, scientists have also modified the DNA of plants so that the plants could fend off insects. In order to accomplish this, scientists inserted a "poison" gene into the DNA of the plant. These are called Bt crops. Bacillus thuringiensis (Bt) is a type of soil-dwelling bacteria that produces a protein that is toxic to many insects. Bt crops have been engineered to produce the Bt toxin in the plant itself. When certain insects attack these genetically modified plants, they take a bite of the plant, and their stomachs explode. Is it a coincidence that many of our children suffer from stomach issues? These toxins cannot be washed off the corn because they are physically in the corn.

These two methods of pest reduction and weed reduction produced a new strain of foods that the human body has never been exposed to. How do we know if the "poison gene" introduced in our food supply is poisonous to humans? When GMO foods were first introduced, the FDA (Food and Drug Administration) determined that they were "substantially equivalent" to conventionally produced food, and the foods were allowed into grocery stores without even a label designating them as genetically modified. The FDA has allowed humans to become a huge genetic experiment without having substantial, third-party studies done to certify the safety of these foods. At the writing of this book, over 60 countries have already required GMO labeling, but the United States is not one of those countries.

The FDA is responsible for monitoring our food supply for safety. It publishes a website that lists pesticides that are used on crops. In 2016, the website listed Bt corn (GMO corn) as a pesticide. Many of us feed this pesticide to our children daily in the form of popcorn, corn tortillas, canned and frozen corn, corn on the cob, and as filler in hundreds of other products.

Over 2,000 studies have been conducted showing that GMO foods are safe for human consumption, although few of these studies came from independent sources. Most can be linked to large companies that stand to gain from increasing GMO crop production. Many studies discredit GMO foods claiming there are significant immune system, digestive and infertility problems associated with a diet that includes GMO foods. Dr. Judy Carman recently performed a peer-reviewed scientific study on 168 just-weaned piglets. She chose pigs because they have a similar digestive system to humans and because some of the investigators had been observing reproductive and digestive problems in pigs fed GMO crops. The study showed that male pigs fed a GMO diet are four times more likely to have severe stomach inflammation than the control group and female pigs have increased fertility problems resulting from a uterus that was 25% heavier than the control group. Another recent study concluded that it takes our bodies 50 percent longer to digest GMO foods, which can cause digestive issues in our children who already have sensitive stomachs.

Are GMO foods a health risk? This is not about waging war against GMO foods. I don't have the background in genetics that I would need to do that. However, without concrete evidence that GMO foods are NOT a health risk to our ADHD kids, I try to minimize my children's exposure to these foods as often as possible. Our kids already have more than their share of challenges, and they do not need to be human guinea pigs for this massive food experiment that the FDA is allowing to unfold.

Look for products labeled Non-GMO Project Verified or those labeled as organic to avoid as much GMO food as possible. During the elimination diet, your children should only eat organic and non-GMO verified foods whenever possible. You can find these foods in most health food stores and mainstream grocery stores. A few of the larger mainstream grocery stores have even started carrying their own brands of organic and non-GMO foods.

Our food supply has changed dramatically in the last 50 years and not just because of the proliferation of processed foods and fast food restaurants. The quality of healthy foods has deteriorated, requiring us to move to organic foods and use supplements when necessary.

Carrageenan

Carrageenan is an extract made from a red-colored seaweed called Irish moss. It is used as a thickener in cottage cheese, soymilk, almond milk, and yogurt, as well as many other foods. Dr. Joanne Tobacman, MD, associate professor of clinical medicine at the University of Illinois College of Medicine, has published 18 peer-reviewed studies that assert that the type of carrageenan that is used in our food supply causes malignancies and other stomach problems. Inflammation occurs, especially in the gut, which is a major issue for many ADHD children, although your child may not complain of gut issues. Most ADHD children have lived with gut issues for so long that they consider how they feel as "normal." They don't know any other way to feel. I recommend avoiding all products with carrageenan in them.

Organic Foods

I recommend buying as many organic foods as possible, but only when it makes sense. Almost all organic foods are more expensive to purchase. I've got a few tips to help you choose when to purchase organic, which can save on your food bill.

If I am going to peel a fruit or vegetable, I typically do not purchase organic. I am probably peeling off most of the pesticides, if not all of them. I purchase organic when fruits can't be peeled and especially when they are small, which makes them harder to wash and easier to ingest larger amounts of pesticides. Some of these fruits include strawberries, blueberries and grapes. I always purchase organic squash, zucchini and corn (including popcorn) because these are now being grown as GMO crops.

There is a widely recognized "dirty dozen" and "clean fifteen" list produced by the Environmental Working Group each year, which points out fruits and vegetables with the highest and lowest levels of pesticides.

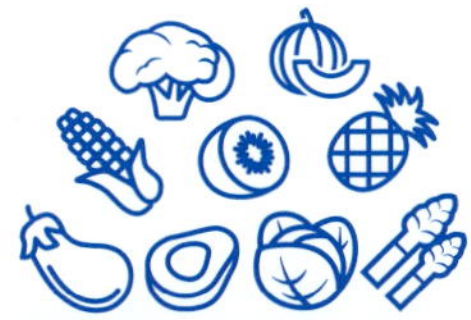

Dirty Dozen	Clean Fifteen
Apples	Asparagus
Bell peppers	Avocado
Celery	Cabbage
Cherry tomatoes	Cantaloupe/watermelon
Cucumbers	Cauliflower
Grapes	Eggplant
Nectarines	Grapefruit
Peaches	Kiwi
Potatoes	Mangos
Snap peas	Onions
Spinach	Papayas
Strawberries	Pineapple
Plus: blueberries	Sweet corn
Plus: green leafy vegetables	Sweet peas
	Sweet Potatoes

Source: Environmental Working Group

"Let food be thy medicine
and medicine be thy food."

HIPPOCRATES

CHAPTER 2

The Eight-Week Program

Changing the American diet from processed food to healthier fare, such as grains, fruits and vegetables, is becoming increasingly important in order to stay healthy. The trick is how to accomplish this feat with our kids. Our kids thrive on continuity. Our kids thrive on control. Our kids thrive on routine. Take away their chicken nuggets? Not so fast!

Alex went to an alternative care practitioner from the Wellness Center when he was eight years old. I will talk more about this treatment in part three on Interventions. One day I had a particularly busy schedule and was forced to take my son with me on a few errands—no continuity, no control and out of his general routine. It was a recipe for disaster. So I did what any self-respecting mom would do. I threw in some snacks and a coveted Ring Pop (these were usually saved for special occasions). We walked into the Wellness Center, and as the doctor was doing the treatment, he noticed the very blue mouth my son had from the Ring Pop. I thought the doctor was going to explode! I received a full-blown lecture on the hazards of dyes and preservatives, and he told me to immediately take all of those out of our diet and start eating vegetables, fruits, whole grains, and all-around healthier foods. I was in a daze walking out of his office. How could I possibly change my son's diet completely and immediately?

Many health food advocates will tell you to go clean out your pantry and get rid of all the "bad" stuff. Don't! The problem with this advice is that you haven't learned about the "good stuff," so you would end up with nothing to eat and would probably resort to grabbing a Ring Pop next time your child demanded a snack. So please heed my advice and take the full eight weeks outlined to work through the detox and diet with your child or entire family. Our kids never do anything fast anyway. Everything is trial and error, slow but steady progress. You should see results by the third or fourth week of the elimination diet, but there is a lot to be done before jumping into this diet.

We will be working with different recipes and menus in order to accomplish a four-week elimination diet. It is critically important to know if your child has food sensitivities and what those are. The only definitive method to do this is to take out the foods with which a majority of children have issues and add them back one at a time and look for reactions to each food.

Before we get to that point, we have to know what foods we can feed our children during that four-week period in order to be successful. I am going to walk you through changing your snacks, breakfast, lunch, and dinner for four weeks. As you go through testing recipes in the first few weeks, be sure to find at least four snacks, two breakfasts, three lunches, and four to five dinners that your child will eat. Don't continue making the recipes because you don't want your child to be tired of the food before you get started with the diet. Make each recipe only once and determine whether your child will eat it or not.

There is no definitive percent of ADHD children that are sensitive to foods. When Feingold first published his program in 1973 he claimed that 50 percent of children tested responded positively to his diet. However, Feingold is only eliminating a small number of foods compared to our elimination diet. We now know that many more children, as well as adults, are sensitive to major food categories such as gluten and dairy. The biggest problem moms run into is trying to eliminate one or two foods, and if there is no noticeable difference in behavior, then they assume their children do not have food sensitivities. However, if the child is sensitive to five different foods, there is little chance that you would randomly eliminate those five foods all at the same time in order to see positive results. Also, if you eliminated two or three of the five foods, you would likely not see positive results because the child would still be eating two or three of the offending foods.

In order to make this as easy as possible, I have broken down the elimination diet into an eight-week program. It is a good idea to read through the entire eight weeks, in order to grasp what is coming each week.

Then go back to week one and accomplish each task as the weeks progress. In order to be successful, there is some timing involved. For example, don't start Week 1 in November, knowing that you will be in the middle of the holiday season and school parties when you are trying to implement an elimination diet. Good times of the year to get through the full eight weeks are January to March, assuming that your children like soups and warm foods. If you are counting on smoothies to keep them filled up and you live in a cold climate, then wait for warmer weather before starting the diet. September through Halloween is also a good time to work through the eight weeks. If you can track their food intake the most effectively when they are not in school, then summer time is a good time to get started. No matter when you get started, you can work through the first three weeks to eliminate toxins, add essential supplements and do some general detox. Once I eliminated many of these toxins, it became a way of life, and I have never gone back to using the household chemicals that are so predominant in our society.

Our kids are typically very picky eaters, so most elimination diets will not work for them. They will simply refuse to eat the wide array of vegetables and salad prescribed by most diets. Through trial and error, I have created a children's version of an elimination diet to get the best results as quickly as possible with the most kid-friendly foods I could find.

Tips and Tricks

Here are a few suggestions to keep you going over the next eight weeks.

1) Find a buddy or form a small group in your neighborhood or at church. The saying that it takes a village to raise a child is an accurate one. A village makes raising a child easier, and it will definitely make the next eight weeks easier. There are so many children with ADHD that if you keep your ears open and talk about your child's challenges, you will quickly find others that have the same problem. Enlist them in this eight-week program. It will be much easier for each mom to make a snack, lunch, or meal and share than taking all this on by yourself.
2) Add fermented foods to your children's diet now. These include sauerkraut, regular or greek plain yogurt (add honey and fruit to taste), and dill pickles (purchase at a health food store to avoid yellow dye). Although your children won't be able to eat these foods once we start the elimination diet, if you feed them these foods now, you

can increase the good bacteria in their guts and start them off on the right track.

3) If your child has had more than one antibiotic a year, it is very possible that he may have a chronic yeast infection. Symptoms of yeast overgrowth can be identical to ADHD symptoms. If your child has been taking antibiotics, it is very important to add yogurt or a probiotic to his diet for two to three weeks before beginning the eight-week program. Also severely limit all sugars including honey and maple syrup for a week and see if his symptoms improve.
4) Cheating on this diet is strictly forbidden. Unfortunately this is not like a regular diet where you keep going if you "cheat". Even the smallest amount of irritating food can trigger an immune reaction for a week or more. This will make it impossible to pinpoint the specific food that is causing these reactions. Enlist your children's help and reiterate to them how important it is not to eat anything, not even one bite of a food that is not on the plan. That is why it is so important to constantly have enough snacks on hand to fill in whenever your children are reaching for something to eat.
5) Sweeteners on this diet will include raw honey, pure maple syrup, and coconut sugar. These are three of the least refined sweeteners that can be used and typically have no added ingredients, although you should still look closely at the ingredient label before purchasing.
6) The only kitchen tool that will be extremely helpful is a high-powered blender or food processor—something that can be used to quickly and easily make smoothies, chop nuts, blend snack bars together, and puree soups. A hot air popcorn popper and a crock pot are also nice, but not necessities.
7) It is important to have your children drink as much pure, clean drinking water as possible each day. The diet will free up toxins from their systems, and they will need plenty of liquids to flush them completely out of the body. The worse your children feel in the first few days, the more toxins are being cleared from the body. Just keep having them drink plenty of water. For a change of pace, they can also drink fresh squeezed lemonade or limeade using honey or coconut sugar as a sweetener.
8) Exercise will also help eliminate toxins as sweating can release toxins through your skin. Be sure that if your children exercise and sweat

that you wipe the sweat off or have them take a shower. Don't let the sweat dry on their skin, or some of the toxins released will reabsorb into their bodies.

9) Bisphenol A (BPA) in plastics should be avoided and totally eliminated during the diet. More than 12 billion pounds of BPA are used every year in plastics such as water bottles and food storage containers. Replace all of your plastic food storage containers with glass containers and purchase a high-quality, non-BPA water bottle to carry around and refill with filtered water.

10) Soups and smoothies are a great menu item for the diet. Once you know your child likes a certain soup, make it in a large batch. To store soup for longer than a week in the refrigerator, let it cool, pour it into glass containers with about an inch free so that it has room to expand and then freeze. Once frozen, close tightly with a lid and store in the freezer for up to three months. If a soup is too thick, such as chili or black bean soup, the glass container will break when freezing. You may need to use plastic for this type of soup, just be sure the soup is completely cool before freezing and allow to thaw naturally before using (no microwaving plastic!)

11) Many recipes call for cooked and cubed chicken. I purchase lots of chicken breasts when they are on sale and package them 2-3 per package and freeze them. Using freezer paper will keep them fresh in the freezer for up to 6 months. When I am serving a chicken dish for dinner, I defrost a pack, put 2 tablespoons of extra virgin olive oil in a frying pan and add the chicken breasts. Cover and cook 8 minutes on medium turning after 4 minutes. Take each chicken breast and cut it length wise to expose any uncooked chicken. Place the breasts back in the pan for 2-3 minutes with the pink side down to completely cook. Remove from pan and cut in pieces.

12) There are a number of grocery chains with which you should become familiar if you are close to a metropolitan area. These include Trader Joe's, Whole Foods, Earth Fare, Wegmans and the Fresh Market. Trader Joe's typically carries the least expensive items, while the other stores each have their specialties. There are also many smaller health food stores in most cities that will carry a variety of organic and additive-free foods. Search out these stores before starting the diet. It is a good idea to visit the stores as well and

spend some time walking down the isles familiarizing yourself with some of the store's products. Items like Coconut Aminos can be difficult to find. (Look for them next to the vinegar). Enlist the help of store personnel. They are almost always willing to help you find an item.

12) Stay away from Acetaminophen, at least for the next eight weeks. More studies are being done linking Acetaminophen use to a decrease in Glutathione production. Glutathione is one of the key substances needed in the body in order to detox. If you need to administer any medicine, stick to products that contain Ibuprofin or aspirin, as long as your doctor is okay with this.

Keep a Diary

Before we get started, let's talk briefly about keeping a diary. We are busy moms, and trying to remember what little Johnny ate yesterday or how he acted, or how he physically felt is not always easy. Keeping a diary will be important as you analyze each day and each food that is reintroduced into your child's diet. It is also likely that you will want to look back to re-analyze this eight-week period at a later time. Set aside a few minutes each night—you will be thankful that you did!

SAMPLE DIARY

Date: ____________________

Breakfast	Lunch	Dinner	Snack

Behavior: ____________________

Physical Symptoms: ____________________

Energy Level Morning ☐

Energy Level Evening ☐

The important parts to this diary will include listing what was eaten for breakfast, lunch, dinner, snacks, and all drinks. Then include a very brief description of behavior, such as "three tantrums today after dinner," "angry and disrespectful at breakfast," or "great kid right before bedtime," and so forth. If you can get a report from your child's teacher each day, include that in the diary as well. Add columns for any physical symptoms such as headache, stomach ache or diarrhea and a column for energy level in the morning and energy level in the evening. You can rate energy levels on a scale of 1 to 5. This will help you draw your own conclusions as the diet progresses.

The columns in the diary include: Date, Breakfast, Lunch, Dinner, Snacks, Behavior, Physical Symptoms, Energy Level Morning, Energy Level Evening.

I had a mom who did a fabulous job with the diet the first week, started adding back foods in the second week and about 10 days later the child said he had a stomach ache. She wasn't keeping a diary and after probing for more information, the child could not say when the stomach ache started. He first said it started at the beginning of the diet and then changed his story a number of times. He simply didn't remember if the stomach ache was only from today, yesterday or a number of days prior. The child was obviously sensitive to one of the foods that had been re-introduced, but we weren't sure which one! We had to start the diet again in order to get the right information. Three minutes a day, writing in a diary would have eliminated this problem and given us the information for which we were looking.

Keep this diary for the full eight weeks. The first four weeks will be a benchmark as we are not diving into the elimination diet until Week 5.

Now let's get started!

Find a buddy or form a small group in your neighborhood or at church. The saying that it takes a village to raise a child is so true.

CHAPTER 3

Week 1: Supplements

This first week we are going to review some of the nutritional deficiencies our kids might be experiencing. If you are just beginning to think that your child might have ADD or ADHD, you might consider sticking your big toe in the water by purchasing various ADHD supplements. After all, if you visit a vitamin store, there are numerous bottles that all claim to help ADHD. My best advice is not to bother with the bottles that claim they can cure or help with ADHD. This is a bigger issue than one bottle can cure. If it were that easy, we wouldn't have 6.4 million kids in our country with this problem!

Note: *Always check with your pediatrician or other doctor before giving supplements to your children, particularly if they are already taking other medications.*

There are some supplements worth adding to your child's daily routine. A functional, naturopathic, or homeopathic professional is a good person with whom to consult. Some pediatricians are also starting to realize the vital roll vitamins play in our children's health. Supplements including magnesium, vitamin D, zinc, vitamin C, B vitamins, omega-3s, and selenium are the main vitamins and minerals that will be helpful to your child's overall health. Probiotics can also be helpful to balance our children's gut bacteria. There are obviously many others that can be added, but let's start with these.

These supplements are not going to "cure" your children. You will hear me comment repeatedly that this is a "building block" approach, and supplements are one of the ways to help your children rebound from the toxins in their bodies. If they don't have the correct vitamins and minerals, their bodies are at a disadvantage as they try to neutralize and eliminate toxins that are ingested. A good foundation to build on is a necessity as we start the sensitivity diet in a few weeks.

All human bodies try to detoxify themselves every minute of every day. Just as we rid ourselves of viruses and bacteria through our immune system, our bodies attempt to rid themselves of toxins through the liver, skin and digestive system. If we are missing vitamins and minerals, as we move into the elimination diet, our bodies will function more slowly to remove toxins as we eliminate foods and reintroduce them.

Magnesium and Sulfates

Rosemary Waring is one of the leading researchers in the biochemistry of autism. Since autism and ADHD are on the same spectrum, we can garner some good information from these studies. She shows on average 85 percent of all autistic children have low sulfate and magnesium levels. Without enough sulfates, the body can't produce sufficient levels of glutathione. Glutathione is an amino acid sometimes called the "master antioxidant" of the human body. Glutathione is a crucial component of liver detoxification and is a major anti-inflammatory and immune defense amino acid. Taking glutathione supplements isn't effective because it isn't absorbed well and your stomach breaks it down before the body sees any benefit. In order for our bodies to make sufficient levels of glutathione, the body must have sufficient levels of magnesium and sulfates. As we increase the level of these minerals in our bodies, glutathione increases, which then helps in detoxification, gut integrity, and digestion.

Some of the symptoms of low magnesium and sulfates include:

- Hyperactivity
- Irritability and impatience
- Aggression and tantrums
- Poor sleep
- Headaches

Although this is a list of symptoms for many different problems in our children, low magnesium and sulfate levels are among the easiest issues to fix. Epsom salt has been used for hundreds of years for a wide variety of health benefits. It is not actually salt but a naturally occurring pure mineral compound of magnesium and sulfate that can be readily absorbed through the skin. You can find inexpensive Epsom salt in a half-gallon container at large retail chains such as Walmart and Target. Look in the soap section.

Twice a week, put two cups of Epsom salt into your children's warm bath water. Make up some fun story about what you are putting in their baths and play some type of game with the new "slippery" water so that they accept the new sensation. Human bodies absorb the correct amounts of magnesium and sulfates through the skin when administered in this way, so there is no need to worry about overdosing. This also avoids the possibility that the gut might be hindering absorption if taking magnesium in a pill form. For an added benefit, pour a half cup of olive oil into the bath if your child has dry skin. Additional benefits of magnesium include helping to calm children down at nighttime, helping with stomachaches, and eliminating constipation. After a busy day, a warm Epsom salt bath is a good idea for mom as well!

If your children are too old for baths, either soak their feet in one cup of Epsom salt three times a week or look for Epsom salt cream that can be rubbed into their skin each night before bedtime. The foot soak is the better choice because it can also eliminate toxins from the body at the same time as your feet are absorbing magnesium.

For an added benefit, add three or four drops of lavender to the foot bath or six to eight drops to the bath water for a calming effect if bathing in the evening. Helpful essential oils for detoxification include grapefruit extract, peppermint oil, and juniper oil. These can be purchased at most health food stores in the form of a tincture. Use the same measurement as the lavender and vary the essential oils to get the most benefit.

Caution: Too much magnesium will cause your child to have diarrhea, so if he has this symptom shortly after starting the magnesium, back off on the amount you put in his bath or the dosage he is taking.

Vitamin D

How much sunscreen do you slather on your children before they go outside in the summer? As moms we feel a responsibility to keep our children from getting a sun burn, both because they are painful and also to keep them from getting skin cancer years later. We are missing vital amounts of vitamin D when we constantly use sunscreen on ourselves and on our kids. Although I am not a proponent of lots of sunscreen, some moms would tar and feather me for suggesting sending a child out into the sun without it, even if only for 30 minutes a day.

Recent studies show that the majority of children in the United States are vitamin D deficient. This can be determined by a simple blood test, so if you ask your pediatrician or alternative doctor to run a blood panel, they should check for vitamin D deficiency. Some of our kids have stomach and intestinal issues, such as leaky gut syndrome. In order to get around this issue, it is easiest to give children the liquid form of vitamin D. Put one drop of a 1,000 IU dosage under your child's tongue at any time of the day. Don't drink anything for a few minutes after this to allow for the best absorption. A good alternative medicine doctor will let you know a brand of vitamin D that they recommend. Be sure that it is a liquid and not a pill.

Zinc Picolinate

There are a number of types of zinc including sultrate, citrate, gluconate, and picolinate. Zinc picolinate is one of the easiest forms for our bodies to absorb. According to the *Handbook of Minerals as Nutritional Supplements*, the recommended dose of zinc picolinate (the best form of zinc to take) is 11 milligrams for all ages.

Zinc Picolinate Daily Recommendation (preferred form of zinc)

All Ages	**11 milligrams**

I find zinc picolinate at Earth Fare, but you can also find it online at a number of different websites. Zinc is one of the body's most necessary minerals for a properly functioning immune system.

Vitamin C

Vitamin C is required by our immune systems in order to fight off bacteria in our environment that we are constantly exposed to. If your child regularly eats fruits and vegetables and has less than a couple of colds or sicknesses each year, then your child probably doesn't have a vitamin C deficiency. Otherwise, it is time to start feeding your child more vitamin C.

The best way to do this is by drinking your Vitamin C without the added sugar that usually is part of these drinks. In a glass container add 3 cups of water, squeeze 1 lemon or 1 lime into the water (filtering any seeds), add 3 tablespoons of honey, stir well and enjoy a very refreshing lemonade or limeade. The juice from one lemon provides roughly 30–40 mg of Vitamin C which is close to 100% of the RDA for children up to the age of 13. The juice from one lime provides roughly 20–30 mg of Vitamin

C which, along with other foods your child is eating, should also be enough to meet the RDA each day.

If your child won't drink lemonade or limeade, Vitamin C supplements are sold in a powder form, pill, or liquid. Stay away from the gummy version because most gummies have dyes, preservatives, and sugar in them, which should be avoided and are not permitted on the elimination diet. The recommended daily intake by the US Food and Nutrition Board of the Institute of Medicine ranges from 15 milligrams to 65 milligrams depending on age. See the table for details.

Vitamin C Daily Recommendation

Ages 1–3	15 milligrams
Ages 4–8	25 milligrams
Ages 9–13	45 milligrams
Ages 14–18 (girls)	65 milligrams
Ages 14–18 (boys)	75 milligrams

Vitamin B Complex

B complex usually consists of a range of vitamins including folate or folic acid (B9), niacin, biotin, thiamin, B6, B12, and riboflavin. Folate plays a key role in building DNA, which forms our genetic blueprint. All of the B vitamins work together to support nervous system and brain health. It is best to choose a vitamin B complex made especially for children. Not many drug stores or vitamin stores carry any variety of these, so your best bet is to shop online for this product and pay attention to the reviews.

Omega-3

Omega-3s have become the rock star of supplements over the past 10 years. They are essential fatty acids necessary for healthy brain function. Only moderate improvements in ADHD have been recorded during omega-3 children's studies. However, it is worth adding this supplement to your child's diet, not to improve ADHD symptoms, but to provide your child's brain with what it needs to function at an optimal level. Many of these supplements don't taste great, so pay attention to the reviews if you are purchasing online. Also, stay away from giving omega-3 or B vitamins at nighttime. They increase brain activity and can make a restful sleep harder for your child. Administering at breakfast is the best approach. If you choose a gummy version of omega-3, be sure there are no dyes in it and also no sugar. Salmon and nuts are two of the best sources of omega-3's that are both included in the diet.

Selenium

Selenium is a trace mineral that plays a key role in metabolism. One brazil nut contains approximately 100 percent of the recommended intake of this mineral for children. Instead of taking a supplement, try to convince your child to eat one brazil nut each day. Raw is best, but roasted and salted will be fine if that is what they will eat. More is not better in this case because selenium toxicity can be a problem if too much is ingested. If your child refuses to eat brazil nuts, take about 10 nuts and chop them into small pieces and add them to the granola recipe I've included.

Probiotics

Gut health has become an increasing concern as more studies link poor gut health to immune system dysfunction and immune system dysfunction is then linked to many different diseases, including ADHD. If your child has stomach aches, constipation or diarrhea on a regular basis, you may consider adding a high quality probiotic to his diet.

Lead

As we try to add supplements, there are some metals that we need to be sure are not poisoning our children. One of the major offenders that may need to be removed is lead. Even though much of the old lead paint once used on school and home walls is gone, there are many other ways to ingest lead. If you are at the doctor's office doing testing for low levels of certain vitamins and minerals, be sure to test for high levels of lead. Your child's lead concentration in his blood should be under 10 micrograms per deciliter. If it is more than that, your doctor should be able to prescribe medical treatment to lower the levels of lead.

Week 1 To-Do List

- ☐ Ask your doctor—whether it is the pediatrician, functional, naturopathic, or homeopathic doctor—to verify the correct dosages of all supplements for your child.
- ☐ Go shopping for supplements or purchase them online and begin giving them to your children. Visit my website at LindaArtis.com for recommended brands.
- ☐ Make notes in your diary.
- ☐ For the next three weeks, before the elimination diet starts, feed your child dill pickles (without yellow dye), and plain greek yogurt with honey and fruit at least a couple times each week. This will help settle his digestive system before starting the diet.
- ☐ Optional, but recommended: get a blood test to determine deficiencies in vitamin D, magnesium, zinc, vitamin C, vitamin B6, vitamin B12, folate, lead and anything else the pediatrician recommends.

Shopping List

- ☐ Plain Epsom salt (add two cups in bath water twice a week)
- ☐ Purchase 2-3 essential oils (lavender, grapefruit extract, peppermint oil or juniper oil) to put in the bath
- ☐ Vitamin D (1,000 IU liquid drops; give each child one drop per day)
- ☐ Zinc picolinate (give each child one 10 mg tablet once per day)
- ☐ Vitamin C make 3 cups of lemonade or limeade each day for your child to drink.
- ☐ Children's vitamin B complex (follow dosage instructions on label)
- ☐ Children's omega-3 supplement (follow dosage instructions on label)
- ☐ Brazil nuts (give each child only ONE per day)
- ☐ Optional Probiotic (follow dosage instructions on label)

According to the U.S. President's Cancer Panel Report, there are about 80,000 chemicals in commercial use in the United States, but only about 2% of those have been assessed for their safety. "The American people—even before they are born—are bombarded continually with myriad combinations of these dangerous exposures."

CHAPTER 4

Week 2: Chemicals Around the House

Before implementing the elimination diet, work around the edges a bit and clean up some of the toxins hanging around the house unnoticed. We will also do some grocery shopping to prepare for the elimination diet this week.

Common Household Toxins

Dishwasher Detergent

Although most modern dishwashers have an excellent rinse cycle, it is still possible that some of the harsh chemicals in dishwashing detergents are left behind as a residue on our plates and utensils, and a small percentage of these toxins might make it into our bodies. Next time you purchase this product, choose something "free and clear." There are a number of these products on the market today for a small additional cost, and in my experience they work just as well as the non-free-and-clear products. Seventh Generation is one brand sold throughout the United States. Why not play it safe and make the change? You will typically be eliminating chlorine, phosphate, and petroleum-based ingredients and dyes. Free-and-clear products are also usually biobased, so they are better for the environment—an added bonus!

Laundry Detergent

Same as dishwasher detergent—pick something "free and clear" without any dyes or artificial scents. If you use a pre-wash spray, also look for something free and clear and skip the fabric softener or dryer sheets. Your kids really don't care if their fabric is soft or not! That's just more chemicals to put on their skin each day. If you like the way fabric softeners reduce cling and make your clothes feel soft, choose a wool dryer ball instead.

Cleaning Sprays

I ran across a great company called Norwex not too long ago. The company is based in Norway and offers all-natural cleaning products. My very favorite are the microfiber cloths. They are expensive but are very durable. The cost of these cloths will be offset by no more purchases of window cleaners and other cleaning supplies. I use microfiber cloths to wash windows and mirrors. They are also a great deal easier to use than a chemical cleaning solution and give better results. Simply wet one cloth with hot water, squeeze out the excess, and wipe down the mirror. Then take the dry cloth and dry the mirror. Perfectly clean with no streaks and no lint every time! I have tried other microfiber cloths for this purpose, but none have worked as well as my Norwex cloths!

Floor and Carpet Cleaners

I still used a Swiffer for my floors until very recently! I had been meaning to go to the store and purchase a more traditional mop—wet it, squeeze it, mop up, and rinse it. Not too long ago, someone suggested the perfect solution. Purchase microfiber cloths at the dollar store or some other low-cost outlet type of store. They should be 10-by-10 inches in size or something close to that. Put one of these on the end of the Swiffer handle and use a spray bottle to dampen it with water. Then clean the floors. Halfway through, take it off, turn it over, spray it again with water, and finish the floors. When done, clean any large debris off of the cloth and throw it in the washing machine.

Carpet Cleaning

I do have a carpet steaming company come and clean my carpets occasionally. Have you seen the companies that actually have the word "chem" in the company name? Please don't knowingly put chemicals on your carpet to clean them. Find a company that uses a water-based, steam-cleaning solution for carpet.

Bathroom Disinfectants

My honest opinion is you just don't need these. Many moms may disagree, and if you can't live without your bathroom disinfectants, then don't. This is about getting as many toxins out of your life as possible, while understanding that we will never get all toxins out of our lives. I use water, paper towels, gloves, and a toilet brush to clean around the commodes and Magic Erasers to clean the sinks and tubs. No harsh cleaners in my bathrooms. My opinion is that if somehow I have left a few germs in my bathroom, that is substantially better than leaving a bunch of chemical residues in my bathroom. Again, if this doesn't work for you, don't get stuck on it, just move on to the next suggestion.

Toothpaste

Toothpaste is an obvious offender since kids always swallow at least some of it every time they brush. Look for brands that have eliminated dyes and preservatives. If a toothpaste is red and blue, it is a good bet that dyes are in it. There is a long running debate in our country over the use of fluoride and I don't plan on getting in the middle of it! For this elimination diet, please purchase a tube of fluoride-free, dye-free, preservative-free toothpaste. I use Tom's of Maine, but the Feingold Food List has others that are also okay to use. Once you have completed the elimination diet, you can add back fluoride toothpaste and check for any reactions or sensitivities. Be careful not to add back any dyes or preservatives.

Soap and Shampoos

Purchasing all-natural soap is easy to do. There are many varieties online and in higher-end grocery stores. Stay away from the dyes and read ingredients to see if the fragrance is from a natural source.

Hand Sanitizers

Throw away all hand sanitizers. Slathering our children's hands with chemicals multiple times each day is a terrible idea. Not only will the skin absorb these chemicals, but also some of it will be ingested as they eat various finger foods. Fifty years ago there was no such thing as hand sanitizer, and I don't remember getting sick that often. Have your children wash their hands with natural soap before meals. Some new research even suggests that if children are exposed to more bacteria when they are young, their immune systems will be stronger as they mature. After all, didn't your grandmother approve of you eating dirt when you were a kid? Her only rule was to wash up before dinnertime!

Candles and Air Fresheners

For now, eliminate all plug-in air fresheners and don't light any candles. Some candles have scents to which children are sensitive, and the same goes for air fresheners. Don't spray any air fresheners in the bathroom or around the house.

Summary

These are the main offenders in and around our house. Of course, there are thousands of other products marketed, and we can't review all of them. The bottom line is to replace the items mentioned above if at all possible and pay attention to any other products that you use frequently and look for alternatives that are less toxic.

Elimination Diet Snacks

Next week we will start experimenting with snacks that your child will eat while on the elimination diet. Starting the diet with at least three to four go-to snacks will help ensure compliance with the entire diet, especially when your child is hungry and needs something quick to eat. We will make these snacks next week, so have ingredients from the Snack Recipes Shopping List on page 57 handy to make the process go more quickly. I would suggest that you start with granola bars, oatmeal balls and sunflower bars. However, if you are sure that your child will not eat one of these three recipes, choose a different one. There are other snacks listed later on, such as fruits, vegetables, and organic potato chips that are allowed on the diet as well.

You'll need some additional items to have available for the entirety of the diet, so check in your cupboard and purchase any from the Organic Stock-the-Pantry Shopping List on page 57 that you don't already have. Be sure to purchase as many spices as possible that are organic. Spices last a long time, and spending a little more on these will help in the long run. Stay away from spices that say "all natural." This doesn't mean anything and is just a way to charge more for regular spices that are not organic.

Week 2 To-Do List

- ☐ Eliminate as many toxins as possible from your home.
- ☐ Make notes in your diary.
- ☐ Go shopping for some grocery and other items to prepare for Week 3.

Toxin-Free Home Shopping List

- ☐ Free and clear dishwasher detergent
- ☐ Free and clear laundry detergent
- ☐ Microfiber clothes
- ☐ Swiffer or similar mop without the refills
- ☐ Magic Erasers
- ☐ Dye-free and fluoride-free toothpaste
- ☐ Dye- and synthetic fragrance-free soap and shampoo
- ☐ All-natural sunscreen

Snack Recipes Shopping List

- ☐ Raw pecan pieces (2 cups)
- ☐ Raw sunflower seeds (2 cups)
- ☐ Raw pumpkin seeds (2 cups)
- ☐ Sunflower butter (no added sugar)
- ☐ Gluten-free oats (quick cooking, no more than five minutes)
- ☐ Cashew butter (no added sugar)

Organic Stock-the-Pantry Shopping List

- ☐ Sea salt
- ☐ Black pepper
- ☐ Cayenne pepper
- ☐ Onion powder
- ☐ Garlic powder
- ☐ Paprika
- ☐ Oregano
- ☐ Cumin
- ☐ Chili powder
- ☐ Ground ginger
- ☐ Ground cinnamon
- ☐ Ground sage
- ☐ Natural vanilla extract (not vanillin)
- ☐ Raw honey
- ☐ Pure maple syrup
- ☐ Dijon mustard (check the label to make sure there is no added sugar)
- ☐ Raw apple cider vinegar
- ☐ Extra-virgin olive oil
- ☐ Unprocessed coconut oil (Nutiva is a good brand)
- ☐ Coconut aminos
- ☐ Coconut aminos Teriyaki Sauce
- ☐ Ground flax seeds (one bag, I like Nutiva)
- ☐ Ground hemp seeds (one bag, I like Nutiva)

The EPA sets strict standards for approximately 90 different types of contaminates that can be found in drinking water. However, levels of a widely used class of industrial chemicals exceed federally recommended safety levels in public drinking water supplies for 6 million people in the United States.

August 2016 study by Harvard T.H. Chan School of Public Health and the Harvard John A. Paulson School of Engineering and Applied Sciences

CHAPTER 5

Week 3: Drinking Water

Before we jump into what to eat, it is important to spend some time on what to drink and specifically what water to drink.

Let's start with bottled water. Don't drink it, especially not while on the elimination diet. Your child might have a reaction to the plastic bottles, which can give off toxins, especially if the bottle has been in the sun. I keep a BPA-free water bottle at the ready for each child to take with them if they will be out of the house for any length of time. Plus this can save lots of money in the long run!

Next, we need to fill up that BPA-free water bottle with chemical-free water. The quickest and least expensive way to do this is to purchase a pitcher with a built-in charcoal filter. This will take some of the worst offenders out of the water, such as chlorine. Many of these pitchers are plastic, and we don't want our clean, filtered water sitting in a plastic container with BPA or BSA. I filter my water and then store it in a glass pitcher. An even better choice is to purchase and install an under-the-sink water filtration system so that all water coming out of the kitchen sink is filtered. Lastly, there are expensive, but very effective whole-house water purification systems that can be installed. In my opinion, the best solution is a carbon filter with reverse osmosis.

Another easy thing to do is to visit your local hardware store and purchase a filtered showerhead. This is a $20 to $40 expense and will filter all the chlorine and some other chemicals out of your shower water. It is easy to unscrew your old showerhead and simply screw the new one on. Most of our kids in elementary school are still taking baths, but I still recommend this to everyone I talk to. Even adults could use fewer chemicals in their lives!

Elimination Diet Snacks

This week is snack-testing week, so let the cooking begin. I would suggest making three different snack recipes and letting your children taste test them. You should have already purchased the ingredients last week for these snacks. Offering choices and letting them decide which ones they like best is always easier than presenting them with one option and hoping they like it. Skip to the snack section to find recipes for this initial testing. Once you know if your child likes something, don't fix it again until Week 5 when we start the diet. Many children will tire of a food quickly, especially if they don't love it. We don't want them to stop eating something before we even get started!

Week 3 To-Do List

- ☐ Address your filtered water options for drinking and showering.
- ☐ Taste test three snack recipes and find out which ones your child likes. (Recipes begin on page 67.)
- ☐ Make notes in your diary.
- ☐ Go shopping for Week 4 food testing, when you'll try out some smoothies, breakfasts, and lunches.

Grocery List for Smoothies

- ☐ Unsweetened flax milk or unsweetened coconut milk (be sure there is no carrageenan in the ingredients)
- ☐ Bananas, organic pears, mango, or canned pineapple (freeze any of these or purchase them already frozen for smoothies)

Grocery List for Breakfast Items

- ☐ Nitrate/nitrite free bacon
- ☐ Organic rice cereal or organic barley cereal (no added ingredients)
- ☐ Hash browns with organic potatoes the only ingredient (Cascadian is a great brand)
- ☐ Plain or Salted Rice cakes

CHAPTER 6

Week 4: Final Preparation for the Diet

This is the week to get all your shopping done for the start of the diet. Make snacks for the first week. Clean out the pantry and cabinets of all offending foods that your child could easily grab and eat while you are not looking. By the end of the week, nothing should be available to eat other than the foods listed in the following section.

This week try out a few breakfast items to make sure you have identified at least two breakfasts that your child will eat. Try cereal, oatmeal, hash browns, bacon, and anything else listed in the breakfast section. Also try out lunch items—sunflower or cashew butter on rice cakes, smoothies, or soups listed in the lunch section. You can serve leftover dinner foods for a nutritious lunch as well. Be sure you have at least four or five dinners that your child will eat and try any out that you are uncertain about.

Below are shopping lists for the first week of the diet, assuming you are using all seven days of dinners. Remove any items that your child will not eat and increase the quantity of the items your child will eat. This is another reason to try all these recipes first. By the end of this week you should know what your child will eat, and the approximate quantity to purchase. If you have to run to the store every day, there is less likelihood that you will stick to this diet. After the first week, you should have a good idea of what is working and what is not working. Create shopping lists for the next weeks based on this information.

Week 4 To-Do List

- ☐ Make snacks that passed the test last week.
- ☐ Taste test some breakfast and lunch recipes.
- ☐ Taste test any dinner recipes that your child may not like.
- ☐ Remove "offending foods" from the pantry, so neither you nor your children are tempted to grab them.
- ☐ Make notes in your diary.
- ☐ Go shopping for next week.

Shopping List

- ☐ Bananas (enough to freeze if making smoothies)
- ☐ Melons
- ☐ Canned Pineapple
- ☐ Pears
- ☐ Mango
- ☐ Lemons
- ☐ Carrots
- ☐ Celery
- ☐ Organic potatoes
- ☐ Onions
- ☐ Sweet potatoes
- ☐ Antibiotic-free whole chicken
- ☐ Antibiotic-free boneless chicken thighs or breasts
- ☐ Nitrate/nitrite-free bacon
- ☐ Flank steak
- ☐ Wild-caught salmon (frozen or fresh)
- ☐ Brown rice pasta spirals (gluten-free Tinkyada is a good brand)
- ☐ Quick-cooking oats (gluten free)
- ☐ Rice Flour (you'll need at least one cup)
- ☐ Raw sunflower seeds
- ☐ Raw pumpkin seeds
- ☐ Raw pecan pieces

CHAPTER 7

Week 5: Elimination Diet

The diet outlined in the following chapters will either confirm food sensitivities or eliminate them as underlying causes of a child's diagnosis. It is worth a few weeks and some extra time and patience to know whether this is an issue for your child. In the end, you will find that your whole family will continue to eat better even after this diet is complete. You will have some nutritious recipes to continue to make, and hopefully cooking, even if it is just snacks or desserts, will be something your children will have learned to enjoy. After all the preparation, we are now ready to tackle the elimination diet.

Unsweetened coconut milk and unsweetened flax milk are the only two milk substitutes that should be consumed for the first two weeks of the elimination diet. If your child won't drink either of these (and mine won't touch them except in smoothies), then stick to purified water or make the lemonade or limeade in the recipe section.

Our kids do not like change and typically are not fans of variety, which can play in our favor when doing an elimination diet. The key to a successful diet is to give them the same thing repeatedly. Breakfast every day can be the same thing. Snacks can be the same. Lunch can be the same. Dinner can vary, but stick to four or five different dinners and then keep repeating them. Be sure you have tried out all the recipes you plan to use to ensure your child will eat them. If you fix a dinner he or she doesn't like, you will be more tempted to provide something that is not part of the diet as a substitute.

Pick a four-week period of time without holidays, special occasions, or trips to begin the diet. It is very hard to stay on this diet unless you are home preparing the food. As mentioned earlier, August, September and October are good months as long as you end before Halloween and January, February and March can also be good months, because most people don't travel during this time and there are few school parties, except Valentines Day. Summer might also work, depending on travel and vacation plans.

Here are the foods that we are eliminating:

- Artificial Sweeteners
- Caffeine
- Casein (dairy)
- Cocoa
- Corn
- Dyes
- Eggs
- Gluten
- High fructose corn syrup
- Nitrates/Nitrites
- Preservatives and MSG
- Salicylates (see list on page 30)
- Soy
- Sugar
- Yeast
- Hundreds of other additives and chemicals

These are the foods that can be eaten:

Meats

Avoid all processed meats such as packaged sausage, pre-packaged burgers and deli meat. Whenever possible, choose anti-biotic free, organic, wild-caught or grass fed.

Beef
Chicken
Fish
Turkey
Salmon
Shrimp
Scallops
Seafood
Pork

Fruits

Organic is best; however, refer to the Dirty Dozen and Clean Fifteen lists on page 35 for further information

Bananas
Grapefruit
Kiwi
Lemon
Lime
Mango
Melon
Papaya
Pears
Pineapple (canned only)
Pomegranate
Watermelon

Nuts

Raw is best. Use the recipe under the snack section to toast seeds and add seasonings. When purchasing sunflower butter or cashew butter be sure there is no added sugar or preservatives.

- Brazil Nuts
- Cashews
- Cashew Butter
- Flax Seeds
- Hazelnuts
- Macadamia Nuts
- Pecans
- Pine Nuts
- Pistachio
- Pumpkin Seeds
- Sesame Seeds
- Sunflower Seeds
- Sunflower Butter
- Walnuts

Vegetables

Organic is best; however, refer to the Dirty Dozen and Clean Fifteen lists on page 35 for further information

- Artichoke
- Asparagus
- Beets
- Broccoli
- Brussel Sprouts
- Cabbage
- Carrots
- Cauliflower
- Celery
- Eggplant
- Garlic
- Green Beans
- Greens (all kinds)
- Lettuce
- Mushrooms
- Okra
- Onion
- Peas
- Potatoes
- Pumpkin
- Radish
- Rhubarb
- Spinach
- Sprouts
- Squash (Summer, Acorn, Spaghetti)
- Sweet Potatoes/Yams
- Swiss Chard
- Turnips

Grains

- Beans
- Millet
- Oats (certified gluten free)
- Quinoa
- Rice
- Sorghum
- Wild Rice

Fats

Coconut Oil
Extra-Virgin Olive Oil
Organic Sesame Oil
Organic Sunflower Oil

Drinks

Coconut Water (no sugar added)
Lemonade (see recipe)
Limeade (see recipe)
Unsweetened Coconut Milk
Unsweetened Flax Milk (no carrageenan in ingredients list)
Water (filtered, not from plastic bottles)

Condiments and Misc.

Mustard (no sugar or preservatives added)
Spices (all except cloves)

Snacks

I have some standard go-to snacks that I always have available. I will suggest a number of recipes to get you on your way to healthy eating. Each takes more time to prepare than purchasing Twinkies at the neighborhood grocery store. I have a busy schedule, so I try to set aside one night each week for "cooking night." Our kids thrive on routines—I know I have said that before—so work the healthy eating into a routine. My cooking time is Sunday afternoon/evening. Before then, I make sure I know what the snacks will be for that week and solicit input from my children. I must have all ingredients on hand by Sunday afternoon, or my best intentions will fall apart. With all ingredients on hand, I can make an amazing mess of the kitchen, and the kids usually pitch in and help. In the end I have two to three snacks to offer during the week that are nutritional yet very tasty, even to the pickiest eaters.

Granola bars are one of my mainstays for snacks. Below is the basic recipe. I have found that my kids will eat this provided they get to determine the ingredients. The most basic ingredients are oats, maple syrup, raw sunflower seeds, and raw chopped pecans. From there everything else listed in the recipe can be up to them. That gives them lots of control and lots of buy-in to this "new" snack. I have two kids. So I will make up the bars with the main ingredients, split it into two bowls, and let each one add their own additional ingredients from the recipe list below.

Granola Bars

3 cups quick-cooking gluten-free oats
1 cup raw sunflower seeds
1 cup raw pecans chopped
1 cup raw pumpkin seeds
1/4 cup flax seeds
1/4 cup hemp seeds
1 teaspoon salt
1 teaspoon cinnamon
1 cup maple syrup
1/4 cup olive oil
1 teaspoon vanilla
1/4 cup cashew butter

Preheat oven to 300 F. Mix dry ingredients. Mix wet ingredients. Combine together, add cashew butter and mix well. Mound bars or balls on a cookie sheet lined with parchment paper. Bake for 18 to 20 minutes, removing briefly from the oven halfway through baking to flatten each bar with a spatula. This will help hold the bar together when it comes out of the oven. After removing from the oven, cool for five minutes and then transfer bars to a cooling rack. Bars will be brittle, so be careful moving them around. Worst case, a bar becomes granola pieces. Granola pieces can be stored in a mason jar in the refrigerator for up to three months.

Variation: *When testing for cacao, add 2 tablespoons of cacao powder to this recipe.*

Oatmeal Balls

2 cups quick-cooking, gluten-free oats
1/2 cup sunflower butter OR 1/2 cup cashew butter
1/4 cup water

Dump oats in a bowl. In a separate bowl, mix sunflower butter or cashew butter with the water. Add this mixture to the oats. Add more water for a little softer ball. Put in the refrigerator to set for a couple of hours before serving. For a sweeter treat, substitute honey for the water.

Variation: *When testing for almonds or peanuts, substitute almond butter or peanut butter for sunflower butter. If your child does not have sensitivities to cacao, dairy, or sugar, add 1/4 cup mini semi-sweet chocolate chips.*

Sunflower Bars

1 cup quick-cooking, gluten-free oats
1/2 cup sunflower butter
1/4 cup coconut oil
1/3 cup honey
1/4 cup ground hemp or flax seeds (or both)
1/4 teaspoon ginger

Microwave coconut oil until melted. Mix all ingredients and press into a pan covered with wax paper. Put in freezer for two hours to harden. Cut into squares. Store in freezer until ready to eat.

Sweet and Salty Mixed Nuts

2 tablespoons coconut oil
2 tablespoons pure maple syrup
1 teaspoon salt
3/4 cup raw cashews
1/2 cup raw walnut halves or pieces
1/2 cup raw pecan halves or pieces
1/4 teaspoon cayenne pepper

Preheat oven to 300 F. Microwave coconut oil until melted. Add maple syrup, salt, and cayenne pepper. Combine nuts and pour coconut oil mixture over them, tossing well to coat. Line a baking sheet with parchment paper and spread nuts evenly on the baking sheet. Bake for 20 minutes. Remove from oven and sprinkle with cayenne pepper and additional salt to taste. Cool.

Nut Butter Bananas

Slice a banana into a bowl. Mix 2 tablespoons of cashew butter or sunflower butter with 1 tsp honey and then mix with the banana. Sprinkle with walnuts and enjoy.

Roasted Nuts

1 tablespoon coconut oil
1 teaspoon Basic Seasoning (see page 71)
1 teaspoon sea salt
2 cups raw unsalted sunflower or pumpkin seeds

Preheat oven to 275 F. Microwave coconut oil until melted. Mix all ingredients together and spread evenly on cookie sheet. Bake for 10 minutes, stir, and bake for an additional 10 minutes. Cool.

Lemonade or Limeade

3 cups water
1 lemon or lime
3 tablespoons honey

Pour water into a pitcher. Squeeze the lemon or lime into the pitcher making sure to filter out any seeds, add honey and stir.

Melon Pops

Blend 2-4 cups watermelon or cantaloupe in blender and pour into an ice pop mold or Dixie cups with a spoon or popsicle stick inserted in the middle. Freeze and eat.

Veggies

Spread cashew butter on celery sticks. Dip carrots, celery, broccoli, and cauliflower in organic hummus (no preservatives or sugar added –Roots is my favorite brand).

Fruits

Fruit always makes a great snack. Stick to melons (such as watermelon, cantaloupe and honeydew), bananas, pears, mango, kiwi, and canned pineapple (no fresh pineapple because it is high in salicylates).

Nuts

A handful of roasted sunflower seeds, pumpkin seeds, pecans, walnuts, or a brazil nut are always nutritious snack options.

Organic Potato Chips

If you do not have extra time to cook or if you run out of snacks toward the end of the week, have a bag or two of organic potato chips on hand. Chips should never have more than three ingredients: organic potatoes, oil (not soybean), and salt. During this elimination diet, stick to the brands that have sea salt and pass on the other varieties such as sour cream and onion or BBQ. These will have ingredients that are not allowed on the diet.

Breakfast

There are a number of cereals on the market now that are single-ingredient cereals. My kids' favorite is organic rice cereal. The ingredient is "organic rice"—that's it. Most health food stores stock single grain cereals, as well as various cream of rice or organic quinoa products. Add a tablespoon of honey or maple syrup and use either unsweetened coconut milk or flax milk. Add a banana on top or another fruit (see list of acceptable fruits in the Snack Section), and your child will have an excellent breakfast for the next two weeks. If you have more time in the morning, try hash browns and nitrite/nitrate-free bacon. My kids still beg me to make these in the morning.

Hash Browns

16-ounces organic shredded potatoes
3 tablespoons olive oil
2 teaspoons Basic Seasoning (recipe on page 71)

Some stores sell frozen hash browns with "organic potatoes" as the only ingredient, no added fillers or preservatives. Cascadian is one of these brands. If you can't find these, try shredding your own organic potatoes. In a pan over medium heat, pour olive oil in the bottom and then sprinkle one teaspoon of Basic Seasoning evenly into the oil. Dump hash browns into the pan and smash them down with a spatula. Sprinkle one teaspoon of Basic Seasoning evenly on top. Cover and cook on medium for 10 minutes. Flip hashbrowns over with a spatula and cook an additional 10 minutes until golden brown.

Basic Seasoning

2 tablespoons salt
1 tablespoon ground black pepper
1 tablespoon onion powder
1 tablespoon garlic powder

Combine all ingredients and store in an airtight container. Make a batch of this seasoning before starting the diet. You will use it in a number of different recipes to add flavor. I typically double or triple this recipe to save time.

Oatmeal Cookies (for Breakfast!)

2 medium ripe bananas, mashed
1 cup quick-cooking gluten-free oats

Preheat the oven to 350 F. Combine all ingredients and drop by the spoonful onto a cookie sheet. Bake for 15 minutes.
These are great right out of the oven but are mushy the next day if heated in a microwave. If you have them left over, put them back in the oven or a toaster oven for a few minutes to crisp them up.

> **Variation:** *If your child does not have sensitivities to cacao, dairy, or sugar, add 1/4 cup mini semi-sweet chocolate chips.*

Sausage

Commercial, prepackaged sausage contains nitrates, nitrites, sweeteners, preservatives and more. Try this easy recipe to make healthier sausage.

1 pound ground sausage from the meat department (not prepackaged)
1 teaspoon salt
1/2 teaspoon pepper1/2 teaspoon sage
1/4 teaspoon ginger
1/4 teaspoon cayenne pepper

Mix all ingredients, form into patties, and pan fry until cooked on both sides and in the middle.

Rice Cakes

If your child will eat rice cakes, purchase plain or salted and add sunflower butter and a little honey or maple syrup for sweetness. Cashew butter is a little sweeter and can also be spread on rice cakes.

Lunch

If you undertake this diet during the school year, you will need to have your child help pack a nutritious lunch each day. He or she also has to agree not to exchange any food with other kids, just for this short period of time. If you are not sure your child can do this, consider going to lunch with him or her the first few days if your school allows this to monitor the situation.

Lunch Ideas

Invest in a small thermos for hot foods and soups, including dinner leftovers. Chicken fried rice makes a great leftover lunch. My kids also loved taking the flank steak (see dinner recipes) cut up in pieces in their thermoses. Other meats can be packed in a thermos as well, but stay away from deli style lunch meats, which have lots of preservatives in them.

Other good lunch ideas include rice cakes with sunflower butter (mix sunflower butter with a little honey before spreading it if your child needs more sweetness) or cashew butter; fruit (melons, bananas, pears, canned pineapple, grapefruit); and organic potato chips.

And don't forget to fill up a metal or glass water bottle with filtered water for your child to drink.

Black Bean Soup

1/2 cup finely chopped onion

1 large clove garlic finely chopped

2 tablespoons extra virgin olive oil

2 15-ounce cans organic black beans drained

1 cup chicken broth

1 tablespoon cumin
1/2 teaspoon salt
1/2 teaspoon pepper
1/8 teaspoon cayenne pepper

In a sauce pan, combine onion, garlic and olive oil. Cook 5 minutes. Slightly puree the black beans in a blender and add to the onion and garlic mixture. Add remainder of ingredients and bring to a boil. Reduce heat and simmer uncovered for 20 minutes stirring occasionally. Serve.

Variation: *When testing for dairy sensitivity, top with grated cheese and sour cream.*

Banana Smoothie

2 frozen bananas
1 1/2 cups unsweetened flax or coconut milk
1/4 cup hemp seeds
2 tablespoons pure maple syrup

Blend all ingredients and serve.

Fruit Smoothie

2 cups frozen mango or canned pineapple chunks or 1 cup of each
1 1/2 cups unsweetened flax or coconut milk
1/4 cup hemp seeds
2 tablespoons maple syrup

Blend all ingredients and serve.

Variation: *When testing for cacao sensitivity, add 2 tablespoons cacao to the banana smoothie. When testing for sensitivity to dates, substitute 4 pitted whole dates for the maple syrup in any smoothie.*

My children and I had fun with this recipe after the first week of the diet, when we added back cacao. We used three different fruits, which included frozen bananas, mango, and canned pineapple, and made the basic recipe. We poured out a small "taster" cup and then added one tablespoon of cacao powder to the remainder of the mixture still in the blender and blended again. We poured a second small cup and added a second tablespoon of cacao powder to the blender. We poured a third small cup. Our last ingredient to add to the remainder of the mixture was one tablespoon of maple syrup. At the end we sampled all four and decided which we liked best. That became the recipe I used moving forward. Kids love sampling things and having choices. In the end, both my children liked the smoothie with everything in it. It was more chocolaty and sweeter than the original recipe. Every kid has different tastes, and it is fun to try out this recipe in lots of different ways.

I add ground hemp seeds for extra protein. They have a slightly nutty flavor but not strong enough for your child to taste them. They are high in calories, so add more or less depending on how many extra calories you want your child to have. Many protein powders are made from hemp seeds, so save your money and just purchase hemp seeds. Be sure to avoid green hemp powder. It doesn't taste very good and most of our kids don't like eating things that are green!

Dinner

As long as you have tested these dinners and your children will eat them, I would stick to one week of them and simply repeat them the second week until we start to add back foods. If you can't find enough recipes that your children like, choose as many as they will eat and repeat them for 14 days. Too much variety adds too much complexity to this diet, and we need to keep it as simple as possible.

Crockpot Chicken with Vegetables

2 tablespoons rice flour

1 whole, antibiotic-free chicken

2 tablespoons Basic Seasoning (see page 71)

3/4 cup organic chicken broth (no added sugar)

Vegetables your child likes (carrots, onions, potatoes, green beans)

Set aside the giblets (the stuff inside the chicken), in order to make stock for the Chicken Noodle Soup recipe later. Pour in the broth and sprinkle flour into the crock pot. Add vegetables. Season chicken inside and outside and place on top of vegetables. Cover and cook in crockpot on low for 8-10 hours or on high for 4-5 hours. Save the bones and giblets for soup stock.

Tip: *A Pot Roast can be substituted for the Whole Chicken, if desired.*

Chicken Fried Rice

2 cups cooked chicken cubed
2 tablespoons extra-virgin olive oil
2 teaspoons minced garlic
1/2 cup chopped onion (optional)
1/2 cup chopped carrot (optional)
1/4 cup chopped celery (optional)
1/2 cup chopped mushrooms (optional)
1/8 teaspoon ground ginger
1/4 teaspoon pepper
1 teaspoon Basic Seasoning (see page 71)
1/4 cup water
2 tablespoons coconut aminos
3 cups cooked white or brown rice

In a frying pan on medium heat, add olive oil, garlic, and optional veggies and cook until tender. Add ginger, pepper, seasoning, water, and coconut aminos. Blend in a food processor enough to make the veggies less noticeable if you have a really picky eater! You can skip this step if your child loves to eat orange and green vegetables. Return mixture to pan and add chicken and rice. Fry for 5 more minutes turning once or twice.

Variation: *When testing for egg sensitivity, add two scrambled eggs finely chopped.*

Chicken Stir Fry

2 cups chicken cooked and cubed
1/2 cup coconut aminos teriyaki sauce
2 teaspoons Basic Seasoning
Vegetables – your choice of snow peas, broccoli, onions, carrots

Combine all ingredients except the chicken in a wok or large pan. Cook until tender. Add chicken and heat thoroughly. Serve over white or brown rice.

Tip: *If you choose to make the Chicken Stir Fry and the Chicken Fried Rice within a few days of each other, make a large pot of rice and use it for both meals.*

Chicken Noodle Soup

Giblets and bones left over from the Crockpot Chicken recipe

2 diced onions
5 diced celery sticks
1 tablespoon Basic Seasoning (see page 71)
1/2 teaspoon salt
8 cups water
12 ounces cooked rice noodles
8 ounces cooked carrots (optional)

Place all ingredients except the carrots in a large pot and cover with 8 cups of water. Bring to a boil, turn down heat and simmer partially covered for one hour. Place the entire pot in the refrigerator overnight or for at least 6 hours. (If the pot is hot, place it on a potholder, instead of directly on a glass shelf in the refrigerator) When you are ready for dinner, pull out the large pot and pick the chicken off the bones (discard the bones and the giblets). Combine the chicken pieces and cooked carrots (if your child will eat them) and rice noodles. Season to taste.

Honey Salmon

1/4 cup coconut aminos
2 tablespoons vinegar
2 tablespoons lemon juice
1 tablespoons olive oil
1 tablespoons honey
1 teaspoon black pepper
1/2 teaspoon paprika
1/2 teaspoon garlic powder
1/8 teaspoon cayenne pepper (optional)
1 to 2 pounds salmon

Preheat oven to 350 F. Combine all ingredients except salmon in a small sauce pan and simmer over medium heat for 15 to 20 minutes until thick. Place salmon in a foil-lined baking pan, pour half the sauce over salmon, and bake for 12 to 15 minutes being careful not to overcook. Pour remaining sauce over the salmon and serve.

Taco Salad

1 pound of cooked, shredded chicken breasts or hamburger
1/2 cup water
1 tablespoon chili powder
2 teaspoons Basic Seasoning (see page 71)
1/2 teaspoon paprika
2 teaspoons cumin

In a sauce pan, combine all ingredients, bring to a boil, reduce heat and simmer uncovered 5 minutes until water is absorbed. Serve over lettuce. Sides can include organic refried beans, rice, or black beans.

Tip: *Taco Seasoning can be used for a variety of dishes such as the pork chops below. Save time by making a batch of this and store it in an seasoning jar.*
4 tablespoons chili powder
3 tablespoons Basic Seasoning
2 teaspoon paprika
3 tablespoons cumin

Baked Pork Chops

4 teaspoons taco seasoning (see above recipe)
4 pork chops – 3/4 to 1 inch thick

Sprinkle 1/2 teaspoon taco seasoning on each side of pork chop and place in roasting pan on foil. Repeat for all pork chops. Bake in 400 F oven for 20 minutes or until internal temperature of pork chops reach 160 F.

Taco Bean Chili

1 pound ground beef or ground turkey
1 15 ounce can organic black beans
1 15 ounce can organic navy beans
3 tablespoons taco seasoning (recipe on page 77)

Cook ground beef or turkey in a frying pan, chop into small pieces and drain off grease. Add beans and liquid to the meat. Add taco seasoning and stir until well blended. Heat and eat.

Variation: *When testing for tomato sensitivity, add a 15 ounce can of diced, stewed tomatoes. When testing for corn sensitivity, add a 15-ounce can of organic corn. When testing for dairy sensitivity, top with shredded cheese and sour cream.*

Flank Steak

2–3 pounds flank steak
1/4 teaspoon garlic powder
1 1/2 teaspoon salt
1 1/2 teaspoon pepper
1 tablespoon dry mustard
2 tablespoons coconut aminos
1/4 cup raw cider vinegar
1/4 cup lemon juice
1/2 cup extra-virgin olive oil

Place flank steak in a glass bowl. Mix all other ingredients in a mixing bowl and pour over the steak, being careful to coat the entire steak. Close bowl tightly with a lid and place in the refrigerator for 12 to 24 hours. Remove steak from bowl and discard liquid. Place in a broiler pan and broil in the oven or cook on a grill for 5 minutes on each side to an internal temperature of 145 degrees. Be careful not to overcook, or it will be tough.

Chicken Pasta

2 cups cooked, cubed chicken
12 ounces cooked rice pasta (Tinkyada is my favorite brand)
1/4 cup coconut aminos

Combine all ingredients and place into a glass bowl. Cover tightly with a lid and marinate for 12 to 24 hours in the refrigerator. Heat in a sauce pan or in the microwave before eating.

Vegetables and Salads

If you are a mom who needs to serve a vegetable at every meal, try roasting organic summer squash, cauliflower, or broccoli in the oven. Simply coat with extra virgin olive oil, sprinkle with Basic Seasoning, and arrange on a cookie sheet to bake for 20 minutes in a 350° F oven.

A salad will also work. However, you must stay away from salicylates such as cucumber, tomato, and peppers, and either use oil and vinegar on the salad or use one of the recipes below.

Try a lettuce wedge with the Basic Dressing or Caesar Dressing below and crumbled nitrate/nitrite-free bacon.

Basic Dressing

1/2 cup raw apple cider vinegar
3/4 cup extra-virgin olive oil
1 tablespoon honey
1 tablespoon dijon mustard
1/4 teaspoon salt
1/4 teaspoon black pepper

Mix and enjoy on any salad. Store at room temperature for up to a month.

Caesar Dressing

1 teaspoon garlic powder
1/4 teaspoon salt
1/4 teaspoon black pepper
1 tablespoon Dijon mustard
1 tablespoon raw apple cider vinegar
1 tablespoon lemon juice
1/2 cup extra-virgin olive oil

Blend all ingredients in a food processor and store in the refrigerator.

Oven-Crisp Potato Wedges

1 1/2 pounds organic small red potatoes
1 tablespoon extra-virgin olive oil
1 tablespoon finely minced garlic
1/2 teaspoon salt
1/2 teaspoon paprika
1/4 teaspoon pepper

Preheat oven to 450 F. Lightly coat a baking sheet with olive oil. Mix all ingredients and spread onto the baking sheet. Bake 20 minutes stirring once after 10 minutes.

Alternative: *It is okay to look in the frozen foods section of a health food store for organic french fries. Just be sure the ingredients are "organic potatoes."*

Baked Sweet Potato Fries

3 large sweet potatoes
3 tablespoons extra-virgin olive oil
2 teaspoons sea salt
1/2 tablespoon chili powder

Preheat oven to 450 F. Cut potatoes into wedges or 1/2-inch strips. Combine all ingredients in a bowl and stir until potatoes are well coated. Arrange on a baking sheet and bake for 25 minutes, stirring once after 15 minutes. Cool before serving.

Asparagus Stir Fry

1 tablespoon olive oil
1 bunch asparagus
1 onion finely chopped
1 teaspoon Basic Seasoning
1/2 pound cooked and crumbled nitrite/nitrate free bacon

Not all children will eat asparagus, but if you are lucky enough to have one that likes asparagus, this is a great recipe. Heat olive oil in a pan over medium heat. Add asparagus, onion, and Basic Seasoning and cook until soft, about 10 – 15 minutes. Stir in crumbled bacon pieces. Serve.

Week 5 To-Do List

- ☐ Start the elimination diet.
- ☐ Make notes in your diary.
- ☐ Go shopping for next week when you'll start adding foods back and watching for reactions.

Shopping List

Purchase everything from week one plus the following items:

- ☐ Raw cacao powder
- ☐ Non-GMO popcorn (Skinny Pop or Kettle Brand Popcorn Sea Salt)
- ☐ Eggs
- ☐ Other items from this week's new recipes

CHAPTER 8

Week 6: Elimination Diet

We have reached Week 6, but don't expect big changes in your child...YET! You may see some small changes this week, such as increased energy or a more calm demeanor, but the ADHD symptoms are very likely still there. We are going to add some foods back this week that cause the fewest allergic reactions. These are cocoa or cacao (chocolate), corn and eggs.

The process for adding back a food item is to give the child as much of this item as possible during the day. As you add back each food, look for physical symptoms as well as behavioral symptoms. When adding back foods, the allergic reactions and food sensitivities you are looking for include diarrhea, stomach aches and gas, any rash or redness anywhere on the body, headaches, or heightened behavior issues. These reactions can start within an hour of consuming the food or can take as long as 24 – 48 hours to appear.

Dr. Doris Rapp's book called *The Impossible Child*, suggests having your child write their name before you feed them a new food. Feed them the food and then have them write their name about an hour later. If a child has a severe sensitivity, sometimes the name will look very different after the food has been ingested. When the child writes his name before the offending food is ingested, the name will look relatively neat. After the offending food is ingested and the child writes his name, the penmenship might include writing backwards, upside down or extremely messy. Not all children will have this reaction, but it is worth trying.

Also look for behavioral symptoms. You will likely not see better behavior or decreased hyperactivity during the first week. However, when you add back a food to which there's a sensitivity, you may experience a behavioral reaction such as wildly running around the house, talking non-stop, or being hyperactive in general.

If you witness any physical or behavioral changes after a food has been added back into the diet, take the food out of the diet, wait two days, and then add the next food back into the diet. Wait until the end of the diet before introducing the offending food for a second time. If you get the same results, then your child has a sensitivity to that food. Keep the food out of his diet permanently.

Day 1 and 2: Cacao and Cocoa

On the first day of Week 6, add back cacao or cocoa powder. This doesn't mean a chocolate bar since that includes milk and sugar. Raw cacao powder is a less processed version of cocoa powder, but it is fine to use either. Be sure there are not any other ingredients such as a preservative or anti-caking agent. The ingredients should read "cocoa" or "cacao" and nothing else. Add back as much of this ingredient as possible on the first day of the week. If there are no physical or behavioral changes, assume your child is not sensitive to cacao or cocoa. If you see any symptoms, immediately remove the ingredient, continue two days without it, and then go on to the next ingredient to be added back to the diet. If your child is sensitive to cocoa or cacao, at the end of the diet, at the end of the diet you can add in carob powder as a substitute and see if this is better tolerated.

Ideas for adding cacao in your child's diet include adding 2 tablespoons of cacao power to the banana smoothie or to the granola bars. You can also heat up Unsweetened Flax milk and add 2 tablespoons cacao powder and honey to taste to make hot chocolate.

Chocolate Bark

8 ounces unsweetened chocolate squares
1/2 cup honey
1/4 cup maple syrup
1/2 cup raw sunflower seeds
1/2 cup raw pumpkin seeds
1/4 cup ground flax seeds
1 cup chopped raw pecans
1 cup chopped raw walnuts

Melt chocolate in a glass bowl for approximately 1–2 minutes in your microwave. In a second large bowl, add all other ingredients and mix well. Add the melted chocolate to the second large bowl, mix well and pour mixture onto a cookie sheet covered with wax paper. Put in refrigerator to cool. Cut into pieces and enjoy. Store in the refrigerator.

Day 3 and 4: Corn

The best way to add corn back is to purchase organic popcorn, such as Skinny Pop or Kettle Brand Popcorn Sea Salt. Be sure all corn added back is organic and does not include sugar as an ingredient. At this point, we don't want to introduce GMO corn into the diet along with the pesticides that come with it. You can also serve fresh or frozen non-GMO organic corn, but remember that you cannot put butter on it yet. Salt or other spices are fine.

Corn chips are fine as long as they are organic and don't include sugar as an ingredient. Also look for organic corn tortilla chips. Use the chips to dip with the recipe below.

Three Bean Dip

- 1 15-ounce can organic kidney beans
- 1 15-ounce can organic black beans
- 1 15-ounce can organic corn
- 3 tablespoons extra virgin olive oil
- 3 tablespoons raw apple cider vinegar
- 1/2 teaspoon garlic powder
- 1/2 teaspoon cumin
- 1/4 teaspoon salt
- 1/4 teaspoon pepper

Open cans and drain. Mix all ingredients and refrigerate. Let sit a few hours or overnight if possible. Stir well before eating.

Day 5, 6 and 7: Eggs

Eggs are a great go-to for breakfast. Be sure to purchase high-quality eggs from pasture-raised chickens; organic is always best. The yolks of these eggs will have a deep yellow color due to the increased vitamins and minerals found in them. If you don't believe it is worth the price, purchase a dozen regular store-bought eggs and then purchase the really expensive eggs, which will usually be about twice the price as regular eggs. Fry up one of each and look at the difference. The dark yellow yolk is a visual cue that you are eating an egg that has lots of nutritional value! The washed-out looking egg is just that—washed out. Cooking up eggs, even the very expensive ones, and hash browns makes a very nutritious meal for about \$2. McDonald's will cost you more than that!

The best way to add eggs back to the diet is to make scrambled eggs and nitrate/nitrite-free bacon for dinner one night or fried eggs in extra-virgin olive oil. Serve eggs for dinner both nights if possible. You can also make omelets with nitrate/nitrite-free bacon and veggies such as onions or mushrooms. Stay away from butter and milk until we add those back into the diet. Here is a good egg recipe to try.

Frittatas

8 eggs
1/2 cup unsweetened flax milk
1/2 teaspoon salt
1/4 teaspoon black pepper
Other vegetables cooked until soft (mushrooms, broccoli, or onions)
1/2 cup cooked and crumbled nitrite/nitrate free-bacon

Preheat oven to 400 F. In a bowl, whisk together eggs, flax milk, salt and pepper. Add veggies and bacon. Pour into a cast iron skillet. Bake for 10 minutes.

Week 6 To-Do List

- ☐ Add back in cacao or cocoa, corn, and eggs one at a time.
- ☐ Make notes in your diary.
- ☐ Go shopping for next week when you'll add dairy, tomatoes and apples back into the diet.

Shopping List

Items from previous week

- ☐ Organic Whole Milk
- ☐ Organic Real Butter
- ☐ Sour Cream
- ☐ Organic Marinara Sauce (no sugar added)
- ☐ Block of cheese (no shredded cheese)
- ☐ Gluten Free Noodles
- ☐ Tomatoes
- ☐ Organic Apples
- ☐ Organic Apple Sauce (no sugar added)

A sensitivity to dairy can result from either lactose intolerance, which happens when a child doesn't have the lactase enzyme which breaks down lactose in the digestive system or a casein sensitivity, which is a different enzyme found in many, but not all, dairy products.

CHAPTER 9

Week 7: Elimination Diet

Now it's time to add back a larger food group. Dairy leaves a child's system in about three days, while gluten can take many weeks to be flushed from the system. Let's add dairy first and then we will add a couple salicylates which will include apples and tomatoes and a substitute if your child doesn't like either of these foods.

Day 1, 2 and 3: Dairy

There are a lot of foods that can be added, but the most important to my family is real butter!

Continue with any of the recipes or foods you have been successful with so far. Then add a glass of organic whole milk two to three times a day and test for sensitivities the same way we have with past foods. If he or she doesn't appear to have a negative reaction, continue for two days with other dairy products by using some of the recipes listed below.

If your child will not drink plain milk, then substitute with as much cheese and butter as possible. You can also try plain organic yogurt (no sugar added) with a tablespoon of honey, a handful of walnuts or other nuts, or a crumbled granola bar stirred into the yogurt. This makes a great breakfast or lunch.

Baked Potato Bar

An organic baked potato with cheese (purchase a block of cheese and shred it yourself), sour cream, and butter is a good option. Sometimes I will set up a baked potato bar as my only dinner item. I lay out toppers such as cooked mushrooms, onions, and nitrate/nitrite-free bacon. The kids love topping their own potatoes.

White Chicken Chili

3 15-ounce cans organic white navy beans or organic great northern beans
1 pound chicken breasts cooked and cubed
1/2 teaspoon salt
1/4 teaspoon pepper
12 ounces organic chicken broth (no sugar added)
2 cups mild cheddar cheese shredded
Sour cream

Combine all ingredients into a large pot and heat thoroughly. Serve with grated cheese and sour cream on top.

Popcorn

Homemade popcorn is a staple in my house for snacks, but my kids won't eat it without butter (dairy). Getting rid of the microwave popcorn bags can save a lot of money, and the Skinny Pop or other popcorn you chose when you added back corn can get pretty expensive! Here is how we make healthy homemade popcorn:

- Purchase a hot air popper and teach your kids how to use it.
- Purchase non-GMO popcorn in the bulk section of a health food store. It is much less expensive than microwave popcorn.
- Use sea salt.
- Use organic or regular butter (not margarine).

Measure out the popcorn based on the air popper directions. Melt the butter in a small dish and have it ready along with the salt. As the popcorn is popping, continue to turn the bowl, pour some butter and salt on the popcorn, and turn the bowl again. This will make sure there is some butter and salt on each handful of popcorn that is consumed. It is helpful to have two people do this together, so enlist your child's help. If you pour the butter, let your child turn the bowl and sprinkle on salt.

If you don't want to invest in a hot air popper, you can go the old fashioned route to make popcorn. Pour a few tablespoons of olive oil in a large saucepan (enough to cover the bottom of the pan), heat it up, add popcorn and cover and continue to move the pan back and forth over the stove until you don't hear any more popping. Add salt and butter to taste.

Day 4 and 5: Tomatoes

Next, we are going to add back two foods high in salicylates, which are tomatoes and apples. If your child does not like one or both of these foods, refer to the list of foods on page 30 that are high in salicylates, and choose foods to substitute for either tomatoes or apples or both.

If your child likes tomatoes, they can add a wide variety of Italian dishes to your dinner repertoire. Get ready for something new for dinner tonight!

Add fresh tomatoes to a salad, or use canned tomatoes, tomato sauce or tomato paste in recipes. Check ingredients to be sure no sugar or preservatives are added.

Spaghetti

Let's do this the easy way and grab a jar of organic marinara or spaghetti sauce. It should not have sugar, cane syrup, corn syrup, or any preservatives in it. If you don't recognize an ingredient as a real food or spice, don't buy it! I use Whole Foods' 365 Organic Marinara. Add some cooked hamburger, cooked ground turkey or cooked sausage (ground from the meat section of the health food store, not prepackaged) and serve over gluten-free noodles.

Mexican Rice

1 onion
2 cloves garlic
2 tablespoons olive oil
4 cups organic chicken broth
1 1/2 cups organic stewed tomatoes
2 cups brown or white rice uncooked (not minute rice)

Finely chop onion and garlic and cook in olive oil until soft. Blend all ingredients except rice in a blender until slightly chunky. Don't let your child watch this, because this mixture looks absolutely gross! Pour into a large sauce pan. Add rice and cook 15-20 minutes until rice is soft. Let sit 5 minutes to absorb remaining liquid.

Day 6 and 7: Apples

To add back apples, serve organic apple sauce (check to be sure there is no added sugar), organic apples cut in pieces, half an organic apple, or take out the core and put sunflower or cashew butter in the middle. Core an apple and bake it at 350° F for 15 minutes with a little honey and cinnamon on top. You might also try heating up a bowl of brown rice and adding a couple tablespoons of apple sauce. It is better than it sounds!

If you are adding back other salicylates instead of apples or tomatoes, be sure they are pure and don't include added sugar, preservatives or any ingredients that don't sound like real food.

Week 7 To-Do List

- ☐ Add back dairy, tomatoes and apples (or your choice of other salicylates) one at a time.
- ☐ Make notes in your diary.
- ☐ Go shopping for next week when you'll add sugar and gluten back into the diet and watch for reactions.

Shopping List

Items from previous week

- ☐ Pure Cane Sugar
- ☐ Noodles

CHAPTER 10

Week 8: Elimination Diet

This is the last official week of the elimination diet, and it is time to add back two major categories of foods. These are sugar and gluten. We have waited until the end of the diet to add back gluten because more children are sensitive to gluten than any other food in this diet. If your child experiences a stomach ache or other physical symptoms after adding back gluten, this is a sure sign that he has a gluten sensitivity. If this is the case, don't despair! There are thousands of products on the market today that are gluten free that cater to a growing population that is gluten sensitive.

Day 1, 2 and 3: Sugar

This week we will start by adding back sugar. There are many easy ways to add back sugar. These include substituting 1/2 cup sugar in your lemonade or limeade instead of honey, choosing a non-GMO popcorn with added sugar like Chik-A-Boom, or try the recipe below, for those with no sensitivity to dairy or cacao.

No Bakes

2 cups sugar
1 stick butter
3 tablespoons cacao powder
1 teaspoon vanilla
3 cups gluten-free oatmeal

In a heavy sauce pan over medium heat mix sugar, butter, and cacao powder and bring to a boil. Turn heat down to a slow rolling boil and cook for 5 minutes. Remove from heat, add vanilla and mix well. Add oatmeal and stir until completely covered in chocolate sauce. Place rounded tablespoons of mixture on a cookie sheet covered with wax paper. Put in refrigerator to cool.

I purchase ice cream occasionally (if your child isn't sensitive to dairy), but be sure there are no more than four to five ingredients. There are some excellent all natural ice creams on the market today that eliminate dyes, preservatives, and other additives.

Day 4 and 5: Gluten

It is difficult to add back gluten without also adding back preservatives, so check ingredient lists carefully. Most noodles are free from preservatives and other additives, so cooking a batch of noodles and adding a little salt and butter to them is a kid-friendly meal. You can also try any homemade cookie recipes, such as sugar cookies. Choose organic white or wheat flour in order to keep any pesticides out of the diet. If your child is sensitive to sugar, substitute honey for sugar or look for recipes that don't include sugar. The internet has a wealth of these recipes.

Day 6 and 7: Other Salicylates

You can start adding back other items at this point, but only add one new item every two days to be sure there are no negative reactions. Try adding three to four oranges in a day. Try three to four handfuls of almonds or three to four spoonfuls of almond butter (sugar and preservative free). You can also try 2–3 glasses of unsweetened almond milk, which you could put in your smoothie instead of flax or coconut milk. Serve a cucumber or green pepper in a salad and check for a reaction. You are also free to add back soy or other ingredients, but again, add back items one at a time and wait a couple days to gauge physical and emotional reactions.

I highly recommend not adding back dyes, preservatives, MSG, carrageenan and other chemicals. An occasional handful of M&M's might be okay, but watch for reactions and stay away from buying a whole bag. If your child does have a reaction, then you will know that dyes are a sensitivity.

On page 93 is a standard replacement list of various items that you may be currently purchasing. Replacing some of your old products with these new products will add nutrition and reduce chemicals in your child's diet.

Current Item	Healthy Replacement	Notes
2% milk	Organic whole milk	Years ago people thought fats were unhealthy. It has finally been recognized that fats in foods such as milk are healthy and can help keep kids from gaining excess weight.
Soy sauce	Coconut aminos	Most soy is now GMO. Coconut aminos are similar in taste although less salty and sweeter.
Cocoa powder	Cacao powder	This is the raw version of cocoa and tastes almost the same. And it's better for you!
Breakfast bars, granola bars	Homemade granola bars	The processed varieties are very expensive and full of sugar and chemicals.
Cookies and candies	Find all-natural candy companies on the Internet	If you can't shake the sweet tooth, find substitutes that do not use dyes and chemicals. Feingold's web page has a number of good resources for this.
Chicken	Antibiotic-free chicken	Almost all health food stores carry this at almost the same price as regular chicken.
Flour	Organic flour	Find organic flour in health food stores to eliminate the wide use of pesticides on wheat.
Taco seasoning	Homemade taco seasoning	If this is a family favorite, make enough to keep in a jar, so it is just as convenient as the packaged version. (See page 77 for recipe.)
Peanut butter	Sunflower butter, cashew butter or almond butter	Although peanut butter is okay, these alternatives can taste better and have more nutrients than peanuts. Most peanut butter also has unnecessary sugar or corn syrup added.
Bread	Gluten-free bread or lightly salted rice cakes	Try peanut butter and jelly on a rice cake. My kids love them because they don't get soggy.
Sugar	Pure cane sugar	Be sure sugar is labeled this way in order to avoid GMO sugar beets.

Week 8 and Beyond To-Do List

- ☐ Add back in salicylates and soy one at a time.
- ☐ Make notes in your diary.
- ☐ Go shopping for next week.
- ☐ Keep up with your new eating habits!

Shopping List

- ☐ All items from previous weeks that haven't resulted in a reaction.
- ☐ More items from the salicylates list (page 30).

Everything Else

By now you may have identified some food sensitivities. If there was a reaction to any food group, this is the time to shop for a couple of good recipe books that exclude that food or multiple foods. There are plenty of good cookbooks that specialize in gluten- and casein-free recipes, as well as sugar-free recipe books.

However, if you have added each of these foods back and not witnessed any adverse reactions, then your child most likely has food sensitivities to dyes, preservatives, MSG, or hundreds of other additives that we have eliminated for the past four weeks. You should be noticing some changes in your child's behavior or at least in the amount of anxiety he exhibits. Maybe you will notice more attention and focus, or your teacher might send home a note wondering if you have put little Johnny on some type of medicine, because his behavior has changed for the better.

Discipline

Some behavior problems are learned, so the younger your child is when you do the eight-week program, the quicker the behavior will change. If you have a child that insists on taunting his brother every day when he walks in the door from school, it is likely that this behavior will continue, because it is a habit. The underlying cause for this behavior may be gone, because you have fixed the food sensitivity or the toxicity in your child's body, but he still has habits that need to be broken.

The next section on discipline can help eliminate the learned habits that are causing your child to misbehave. With the new diet actively working for him, these discipline techniques should be easier to implement. As anxiety and hyperactivity decrease, it will be easier to talk with your child, and he will be more open to living within your family structure.

PART TWO:

Routines and Discipline

CHAPTER 11

Week 1: The Bedtime Routine

This section focuses on how to get our children to behave. Our kids respond differently to rewards and consequences compared to other children. A calm, quiet approach to discipline is important in order to end some of their bad habits, but this is by far one of the hardest approaches to implement. This section is broken down into eight weeks of different disciplines and routines to work on.

It is impossible to tackle all of this at once, and it wouldn't be very effective if you tried. Children need a chance to incorporate new rules and responsibilities into their lives slowly. So we'll implement one new idea per week to keep our children's anxiety to a minimum.

We will spend the first week implementing ways to calmly navigate bedtime, one of our children's most anxious and frustrating parts of the day. Although it might make sense to start with the morning, then afternoon and then evening, it is most important to get children to bed in a calm, quiet fashion. The morning routine, and everything in between, will fall into place if we first successfully tackle the bedtime routine. Let's get our kids to bed with a good night's sleep and then review the other parts of the day in the next couple of weeks.

Sleep

Let's talk about sleep or rather lack of sleep. This issue is problematic for our entire society, not just children. We live on too little sleep and too much caffeine and sugar to help us get through the day. We pass this on to our kids, but they don't assimilate lack of sleep into their day as easily as we do. We get irritable if we are tired; they have temper tantrums. Mix "irritable" and "temper tantrum" together, and you get a nightmare!

If your children can't get up in the morning, THEY ARE SUFFERING FROM A LACK OF SLEEP … and please pretend that I just screamed that at you. No matter what parents tell me about their children not needing sleep, if your children aren't wide awake, bouncing out of bed in the morning, it is because they are still tired. The morning routine will work itself out if you can nail the bedtime routine. In other words, get your child to bed on time, and he or she will wake up rested and ready for the day. Easier said than done? Keep reading…

Kindergarten, first, and second graders need at least 11 hours of sleep each night. Third, fourth, and fifth graders need at least 10 hours each night. By the time children are in fifth grade, they may be able to get by with nine hours of sleep one or two nights per week, but not more than that. There are lots of books and lots of doctors that will tell you how many hours of sleep your child needs. The reality is that if your children are not waking up on their own in the morning, they are not getting enough sleep. I will now climb down off my soapbox.

It is hard for children to change their bedtimes, just like it is hard for adults to change their bedtimes. Sit down and have a very quick discussion with your child when he or she is in a really good mood. It goes something like this: "We are going to change your bedtime from 8:30 p.m. to 8:15 p.m. because we are having lots of fussing in the morning, which means you are too tired. If this doesn't work, we will continue to move your bedtime to an earlier time until our mornings get better, with no temper tantrums and a better attitude." You will surely get a temper tantrum over this, so be prepared to walk out of the room. Ignore all outbursts, ugly words, and anything else your child dishes out. You have already given a consequence for bad morning behavior by changing the bedtime, so don't give any other consequences right now. The goal is to move the bedtime and get your child some extra sleep, not anything else. Be sure your child is in bed by the new bedtime.

This is an ideal time to use some melatonin (see next page) for a week or two until your child's body has time to readjust to this new time.

When a birthday comes around or a new school year starts, children seem to think that their bedtime should change. Don't fall for it! If they are supposed to wake up at 7 a.m. every morning, and they are hopping out of bed at 6:30 a.m. awake and ready to go, then it is time to move their bedtime 30 minutes later. Unless this is happening, there is no reason to ever change a child's bedtime! In addition, children need different amounts of sleep. Just because a child is older than his or her siblings does not mean he or she should have a later bedtime.

Melatonin

Melatonin appears to be one of the safest drugs we can give to our kids since melatonin is naturally produced in our bodies.

Disclaimer: *Don't give any type of drug to your child without first consulting a physician.*

Melatonin is a chemical our body produces as it gets dark out and as the day winds down. If our kids are watching TV or are on their computers or other devices, their bodies can be tricked into not producing enough melatonin. The body thinks that it is still daylight. It is best to cut off any screen usage at least an hour before bedtime. If your child is playing computer games anytime after dinner, there is a good chance he has a high level of adrenaline in his system that is also keeping him awake. Immediately after dinner, wrap up any remaining homework, and then try reading books, playing board games, or cards. Stay away from video games and other devices with screens after dinner.

If this still doesn't work, I have found that most elementary school children will respond to 1 mg of melatonin. More is not better. In fact some studies have shown that taking too much melatonin will cause insomnia. So start out with a 1 mg tablet 30 minutes before bedtime. Once my son was consistently sleeping better for about three months, I stopped giving these to him except sporadically when necessary.

For our family, certain events warrant the use of melatonin:

- When school starts (we use it for about two weeks)
- When daylight saving time starts
- When I have to change a child's bedtime to an earlier time
- After a break, such as Christmas or spring break
- When there is an activity that lasts later than 7:30 p.m. such as Cub Scouts, football, baseball, and so forth. We limit these to one or two activities per week.

If you have more than one or two extracurricular activities a week in the evening, consider dropping the least favorite activity. At the end of the day, a calm, well-adjusted child is more important than teaching Johnny to play soccer, basketball, or football—fill in the blank.

Sample Schedule

Our lives are all busy and very complicated, so the more days you can have the same general evening routine, the better. Make sure the children get their homework finished in the afternoon or immediately after dinner, so it doesn't interfere with the bedtime routine. Here is what our evening schedule typically looks like:

- 5:30 p.m. dinner and clean up
- All children make their lunch for the next day with parent help (more on this later)
- Family outside for exercise if time permits (you will need an alternative during bad weather, such as playing a game, reading, or baking)
- Bath time
- End-of-day checklist (see below)
- 7:45 p.m. in bed and lights out
- 8:00 p.m. asleep (hopefully!)

The routine will need to be modified for days when extracurricular activities are scheduled. As a stipulation of going to the activity, your child must agree to speed up the bedtime routine or forfeit the activity the next week. I would also suggest that you might want to skip the bath on these really hectic evenings. This might be controversial to some, but my opinion is that if a child isn't going through puberty and doesn't stink, skipping a bath one night or even a couple nights a week won't hurt anyone.

End of Day Checklist

Your child should also have his or her own checklist to follow. Enlist your child's help and grab a piece of soap. Write the checklist on the mirror so that no one can forget it. Here's an example:

- Teeth
- Pajamas
- Feed fish
- Pick four things up off the floor and put them away
- 8:00 p.m. in bed/lights out

If you can't stand the idea of soap on the bathroom mirror, then put the schedule in LARGE letters on a piece of paper and let your child tape it to the mirror—where ever he or she wants it! Be sure your child knows to start the checklist that night. For younger children, a chart with stickers might also be useful if your child enjoys that type of thing.

	M	T	W	T	F	S	S
Teeth	★						
PJs	★						
Fish	★						
Pick up 4	★						
8 p.m. in bed	★						

So here's the key—don't ever tell your child what to do again. Ten minutes before it's bedtime say, "Go get your stuff (checklist) done. I will meet you in your room at 8 p.m. If you don't get everything done by 8 p.m., your bedtime will have to be earlier tomorrow night." Say all of this in a happy, excited tone, not a threatening tone (even the consequence part). Then here is the kicker—LEAVE and get out of their way! I can almost assure you that our kids will test the consequence part. That's just what they do. So be prepared to move bedtime 15 minutes earlier the next night. You are in his or her room at 8 p.m., and he or she is procrastinating. You simply say, "I am so sorry your bedtime will need to be 7:45 p.m. tomorrow night. Come hop in bed, and we can try again tomorrow." And then DROP IT. No matter what your child says, change the subject as quickly as possible. Do not say the consequence again. I promise your child has heard you but wants to engage in a battle. It is never good to engage in an argument, but one of the worst possible times for this is right before bedtime.

You must be sure to go through the same routine the next night with a bedtime of 7:45 p.m., or all will be lost. Go through the exact same routine the next night, and most children will get it. If yours is particularly strong willed, you might have to do this two to three nights, but stick with it. Can you imagine how different things would be if you have an easy nighttime routine? It will be worth two or three nights of tantrums. When the night arrives when they meet you in their room on time with everything accomplished, be sure to praise them lavishly. Tell them how proud you are and how responsible they have become. Give them a hug and kiss and then get them to bed.

Once they are used to this routine, you can ease up a little. But decide how much you are willing to let the bedtime slide and go back to the earlier bedtime if your child starts procrastinating too much.

I'm Hungry, I'm Thirsty

Every child has an amazing propensity for procrastination. Just when you think you are done for the day and ready to tuck your child in for a peaceful night of sleep, you hear, "Mom, I am hungry," or, "Mom, I am thirsty. Can I get a glass of water?" There are multiple ways to handle this scenario. When my son does this, I usually call his bluff.

To reduce, or even eliminate, this bedtime procrastination, pick a food your child will eat but doesn't relish, like a banana, a pear, a peach, or a handful of nuts. Pick something that you always have in the house, so you can be consistent. Don't pick something that takes a long time to eat and don't ever provide a food he or she really likes, such as yogurt, granola bars, cookies, or anything with sugar in it.

Seconds before my son is ready to get into bed, he will say in his most whiny voice, "Mom, I am starved and won't be able to sleep unless I get something to eat." I immediately call his bluff. I do not get angry or frustrated, which would escalate this simple request and would let him know that he has already won this battle. In a very calm, easy-going tone, I reply, "If you are that hungry, you can go downstairs and eat a banana. I will go with you to get it." Clearly he does not really want a banana. He wants two things. He wants to procrastinate, so he doesn't have to go to bed and he wants a "snack," which to him includes some type of sugar (in other words granola bars, yogurt, cookies, candy, and so forth).

The key is to have a smile on your face, hold firm, and don't give your child any other choices. A banana or bed—either is fine. Your child will likely pick the banana over bed for the first few nights, which is absolutely fine. Go with your child to get the banana with a smile on your face. If your child thinks he or she has won this battle by irritating you, the battle will continue. If the child doesn't get to make you angry, doesn't get the snack of his or her choice, and only gets to spend a few minutes in the kitchen eating, he or she will tire of this bedtime request within a few weeks or even a few days.

There are other options for end-of-night procrastination attempts. Some parents are successful with the "kitchen is closed at 8:00 p.m." approach. Another option is to work a snack into the evening routine. Unless your child is in a growth spurt and is eating a lot more than usual, it is typically not necessary for him or her to eat before bed. Experts would tell us that eating before bed is a bad habit for anyone, including adults.

The one exception to this is that kids on stimulant medication may legitimately be hungry each night. The medicine dulls their appetites, and they don't eat much during the day. By the time bedtime rolls around, they are starved and aren't making this up. If this is the case, then work a snack or a more substantial food into the bedtime routine every night instead of having it come up at the last minute.

Of course, if they can't get anything to eat, they must certainly be very thirsty right before bedtime. What parent would have the audacity to say no to a thirsty child? After many battles over this, I told my child that after I put him to bed and had left the room, he was responsible enough to get up and get a drink anytime he needed to. He did not need my permission. He did not need my help or my approval (or my attention). If he was thirsty, just get up, get a drink, and go back to bed. I put a small cup in the bathroom for him. The trick to this is to completely ignore them, even if they get up ten times the first night.

He got up a few times the first night, a couple times the second night, once the third night, and within two weeks he was seldom getting up for a drink. In the end, he filled up a water bottle and left it by his bed, so if he really was thirsty, he didn't have to get up. He could just reach over and get a drink! This is a good example of giving our kids a little control. They keep pushing and pushing, but if we are willing to give some of our control to them, sometimes the battle just ends. What he really wanted was some extra attention and without that attention, it was no longer worth the battle.

Tips and Tricks

This tip isn't for everyone, but some children (and parents) will appreciate it. Consider letting your child change into their next day's clothes during the bedtime routine and skip the pajamas. If they do not have to wear school uniforms, most boys wear a mix-and-match assortment of shorts or pants and t-shirts to school. Many girls wear leggings and a tank top and then in the morning can throw a longer shirt over this ensemble for school. This is just one less step for our children to master if they are comfortable sleeping in their clothes. And they really don't look that wrinkled when they walk out the door. I promise! As they grow older and are more concerned about their appearance, they will outgrow this habit, but by then the bedtime routine will be easier.

CHAPTER 12

Week 2: The Morning Routine

Sometimes the weekday morning routine is the hardest for parents. There is a lot going on, and everyone is tired and cranky. Why is it so hard to get kids up and moving in the morning? Please refer to Week 1 for the answer to this question! If you have a happy, well-rested kid, a morning routine is by far the easiest of the day.

If you have not had enough sleep, don't impose a cranky attitude on the entire household. If you can't be calm and happy in the morning, then maybe you should also consider a little more sleep.

If certain chores are accomplished as part of the bedtime routine, then morning becomes much easier. I highly recommend enlisting your child's help to pack school lunches. This is a great bonding experience between you and your child, especially if it is accomplished in the evening when there is less stress and a little more time to let your child take the lead. All the room-temperature foods can be put in the lunch box, and the refrigerated items can be placed in one spot in the refrigerator for easy retrieval the next morning. Depending on the child's age, either you or your child can be responsible for putting it all together in the lunch box, which should take only seconds to accomplish in the morning.

Allow extra time the first week or two of school to get the timing down. No one knows exactly how long it will take little Johnny to tie his shoes on a school day. If you budget two minutes and it takes him six minutes, tempers could get short, and a tantrum will ensue. Waking up early isn't fun, especially the first few days of school, but typically it is necessary!

Alarm Clocks

Today you should go shopping with your child and purchase an alarm clock that is really cool (if he or she doesn't already have one). I am a firm believer in clock radios because alarms that use a song, calming waves, or forest sounds are so much easier on our kids than the loud obnoxious buzzer of some clocks. It is best to place the clock on the other side of the room, so they are forced to get up in order to shut it off.

We are going to get rid of what I call the "wake-up tantrums." All school-age children are old enough to set their own alarm clocks and get up when they go off. If they are getting enough sleep, they should already be awake, but a backup is always a good idea. A parent shouldn't be the backup.

The first part of the morning routine is for our children to get up on their own and take control of their own waking. I want to emphasize that the clock should not be placed next to the bed, and the music needs to be loud enough to be annoying. With the cool new alarm clock, your child will likely get up for the first few mornings on his or her own. This may continue if your child is rested and ready to get up anyway. If he or she is exhausted because you have not yet nailed the bedtime routine, then you may have some trouble. Your child might slip back into an old routine. Be sure to use plenty of praise and smiles every morning your child gets up on his or her own. If your child still can't get to the bus stop or in the car at the agreed-upon time, then the natural consequence is to set the alarm for 10 minutes earlier the next morning. Don't be condescending or mean about it. When it is time for bed simply say, "You had a problem this morning getting out the door on time. I am going to set your alarm clock 10 minutes earlier, so we will have a better morning tomorrow." Reset the alarm clock, and don't say anything else. If there are still problems getting out the door on time the following morning, keep moving the alarm back until your child has the time needed to get everything accomplished.

Checklists

If the checklist worked really well for the bedtime routine, then don't hesitate to use a similar one for the morning routine. A checklist might include the following:

- Get Dressed
- Eat
- Brush Teeth and Hair
- Pack lunch
- Pack Backpack
- Meet at Door at 7:00am

Parents should stay out of their children's way when they are getting ready for school in the morning. Unless your child is too young to get their own breakfast or tie their own shoes, you should go about your own chores or get your own breakfast. If your child needs additional attention in the morning then plan to sit down and eat breakfast with them for five minutes in the morning to discuss any apprehension they have about the day or to simply give them some positive praise and attention. If a child is in 3rd grade or above, it can work best to "disappear" while they are getting ready, like take a shower or take the dog for a short walk. Keep in mind that the first few mornings your child will miss the bus or will not be in the car on time. Plan on this and be happy that he is late. There is no lesson to be learned if he makes it on time the first day. This means you will set the alarm clock back by 10 minutes and give him another chance tomorrow to get this right all by himself, as a responsible, trusted child. No yelling, no fussing, just smiles and assurances that he will make it tomorrow morning.

Some children simply move slower than others, and no matter how much we try to hurry them up, they won't get any faster. I have one child who takes 45 minutes to get ready in the morning and one who takes 15 minutes. Both do the same thing in the morning—one just moves at lightening speed and the other at turtle speed.

I no longer say a word to my children in the morning, other than normal morning pleasantries. I show up to drive them to school, and they are in the car at 7:45 a.m. At ages 10 and 13 years old, they pack their own lunches, pack up their book bags, and do basic chores like feed the animals. Then we walk down to the car together. If they are more than a few minutes late, their alarm clock times will change the next night. I never get into an argument with them in the morning. Our children are already worried about school each morning. They need our support and praise in the morning, so they can start out calm and collected.

Tips and Tricks

If the alarm clock has to be set too early in the morning, then that should impact the child's bedtime. If a child needs 11 hours of sleep and has to get up 30 minutes earlier than usual in order to get out the door on time, then bedtime must be 30 minutes earlier.

As your child is almost certainly going to be late for the next few days, give your boss a heads up that you will be late so that you aren't stressed when your child misses the bus. If you drive your child to school, plan on parking and walking in to sign him in late, but don't be angry about it. If you are happy and easy going, your child will learn this very important lesson much more quickly. The consequence is not that he gets to make you mad or control your feelings. The consequence is that he will be waking up 10 minutes earlier the next day, and perhaps having to go to bed earlier as well, if he is too tired in the morning.

CHAPTER 13

Week 3: The After School Routine

Our kids usually come home from school in bad moods. They have a really hard time keeping it together at school for six to eight hours a day. Many times they have had discipline issues at school. Many schools have different red, yellow and green types of discipline scales, and our kids are seldom on green. I would suggest that school discipline should be left at school, and home discipline should be for home behavior. In other words, when you give a consequence for bad behavior at school, your child is being punished twice, and you start out the afternoon with more frustration because your child knows there is a punishment waiting at home. I think it is okay to give a small reward for a good day, but don't issue a consequence for a bad day. It has already been a bad day, and your child has likely already been given a consequence. Let's not make it worse.

Snacks

Start the afternoon on a positive note. Don't even ask about the day's discipline grade. Your anxiety over your child's behavior at school can taint the entire afternoon and evening if you let it. Greet your child with a smile and a good wholesome snack such as the Oatmeal Balls or Granola in the snack recipe section. My kids' other favorites are smoothies and hot air popcorn. It is an added benefit if the snack is something you can make together. Enjoy just a few more minutes of down time before tackling the next big challenge—homework.

Screen Time

Some parents have told me that 30 minutes of TV or computer time settles down their kids and puts them in the right mindset for homework and if that works for you then keep doing it. I have tried this idea and have failed miserably. I believe screens should be the reward for completing homework. Otherwise, there is no real reason for our kids to do their homework. Many of them, mine included, are simply not that motivated. I think I finally got it right by the time my second child was in fifth grade. He came home from school and unpacked his backpack. I helped him make a snack, or if I was not available, he got something himself. Then it was time for homework. If he completed his homework, then his reward was screen time before dinner or he could go outside and play with his friends. If there was lots of fussing or the homework was not complete, there was no screen time or other playtime. Period. That was the rule. Enforce it just a few times, and homework will start getting done. If this is challenging for your family then add homework completion to the list of rules when you get to Week 5.

Homework

So let's talk about the act of doing homework. Some kids absolutely must have a parent's help to get their homework completed. In elementary school, my daughter (who has ADD), was one of those kids. She just didn't know where to start, and so much of the material confused her. In this case, I had to sit with her and help her get assignments completed.

My son, on the other hand, "faked" not knowing how to do homework, so he could get me to do the same thing with him, but I think most parents can tell the difference. He is an extremely bright child and could easily do homework by himself, but tried his best to get me to do it for him. My best suggestion is to simply not be there when they are doing homework. Be in the other room doing laundry, in the kitchen fixing dinner, or outside watering the plants. Be anywhere except close enough to hear them whining about how difficult the homework is. If it is impossible to do this, then the next best option is to give them 30 minutes of screens if they need your help but 60 minutes of screens if they finish all by themselves. I think it is important to give them some reward for completing the homework, even if you do have to help them—as long as it is complete by dinnertime.

If you believe the homework load is too much for your child, visiting the teacher to discuss the amount of homework and other options is always worth a try. Alex had 15 sentences to write every Tuesday, which he just couldn't seem to write. I asked the teacher to let Alex write five really good, long sentences, instead of 15 short, painful, frustrating sentences. She agreed. I sat down with Alex and asked him to come up with a four- to five-word sentence. Then together we would expand that to a 10-word sentence. I believe he learned more and got less frustrated than with the 15 sentences. Hopefully you will have teachers who are as willing to work with you as ours were. It is always worth it to spend time trying to advocate for your child when it comes to homework.

Tips and Tricks

It is good to have a homework-friendly area for your child to use each day. Let them spread out on a kitchen table or curl up on a sofa or chair if that is their preference. Try to remove distractions, including noisy siblings, if possible. There should be no TV, radio, access to their phone, and so forth in this location. After they are finished with homework, they can have access to screens if that is your agreement.

If they have homework in multiple subjects and don't know where to start, help them decide if they want to do the easy work first or get the harder subjects out of the way. Each child is different, so let them make the final decision.

Let two or three things go this week that aren't a priority. Pick your battles; not everything is worth a confrontation.

CHAPTER 14

Week 4: House Rules

This week we are going to create and publish some house rules. One of the most problematic situations for parents is when our children do something wrong and we have to immediately, off the top of our heads, come up with consequences—when we are boiling mad. This never turns out well. We either go way overboard with a consequence we can't enforce or end up in a screaming match.

Every household should have a list of rules that will be enforced with consequences or attained using rewards. The list should include about five to seven items of your child's most frustrating behaviors. At first, there will be some really big ones, like getting homework done and getting As and Bs in school. Here is a sample of what my first list of rules looked like.

Rules	Consequence
Cannot get a C or lower on a quarterly midterm or quarterly report card.	No computer or iPad for two weeks. Must review homework with parent each night.
No disrespect or tantrums when computer time is over.	No screens the next day.
Not getting off screens when asked.	No screens the next day.
Honor commitments—go to all practices or meetings.	No screens the next day.
Do not use mean words.	Write 10 sentences for each word that is not allowed.
Must eat snack and do homework BEFORE any screens. Kitchen is closed at 4 p.m. until dinner.	
Earn 30 minutes of TV time at night by doing something active outside after dinner for 30 minutes.	

"Screens" include TV, Xbox, computer, iPhone, iTouch, iPad, and so forth. The key to this list is to present it to your child as the law of the land. Your child will likely shrug it off as just another parental attempt to ruin his or her life. Don't get angry, just post the rules somewhere your child can see them and let him or her know the rules are there. If your child can't read, you will need to go over them with him or her. When your child breaks the first rule, have empathy. Say something like, "I am so sorry that you forgot to get your homework done yesterday. The rules say you won't have any computer time today." As the temper tantrum begins and they start into how unfair you are, make a quick escape from the room. Don't hang around to get into an argument. Your child can't have a temper tantrum if you are not present.

As you gain compliance in some areas, other items can be added to the list. Publish the list somewhere that is easily accessible and can be referred to often. My son tore the list off the wall and threw it in the trash. I ignored the behavior and put up a new list after he went to bed. After a few days he decided to ignore the list, but he knew it was there, what was on it, and what the consequence was for breaking a rule. Of course, the key here is to follow through with the consequence. If you think, even for a minute that you cannot or will not enforce the consequence, then impose a different consequence—one that you are sure you can enforce.

The constant mantra in our house is "pick your battles." If there are too many battles going at once, you will lose them all. Nagging erodes the relationship you have with your child. Don't engage in it. It is not necessary. Let it go. If there is underwear in the middle of your child's floor, just let it go. Eventually, this will make it onto the list of items that have consequences. If you decide it is that important, add it to the list, and the behavior will change. If it is not one of the top five to seven behaviors you want changed first, please let it go—just for the short term. If you can't stand the underwear on the floor, pick it up yourself, but don't say a word. Don't groan. Don't appear in the least bit upset. This will be a battle for another day, when picking up clothes is a high enough priority to make it to the list.

Let It Go

Let go of two or three things this week. This goes along with picking your battles. My husband goes crazy every time our son doesn't put his shoes in the designated shoe spot. Personally, I don't think it is worth a daily fight to get the shoes put in the proper location. I would much rather ignore where the shoes end up or move them myself. It is not a battle I am willing to fight, and it is not a high enough priority to add it to the list of rules. On the other hand, I will fight all day to be sure homework is completed. That is one of my battles I am willing to fight. So today think of one thing that really won't hurt anyone if you just drop it, ignore it, forget about it. It's just one less thing to fight about, and our kids have really had enough fighting! And the shoes—when it gets to be a priority, put it on the rules list and attach a consequence, and the behavior will get fixed.

Reasonable, enforceable consequences are one of the keys to calm, effective parenting and happier, well adjusted kids.

CHAPTER 15

Week 5: Consequences

A multitude of books are on the market about how to discipline children. Parents can read about being too strict or being too lenient. We can read about how to give consequences and how to give rewards. We can read about putting kids in time outs or about spanking them. I have personally read dozens of books on the subject of discipline, and they all make me mad. They say things like, "The only reason a child has a tantrum is because he knows you might give in to his demands." I have never given in to his demands, but still I am labeled a bad parent because he continues to have tantrums. Another common piece of advice goes something like this, "Put a list of rules up in the house, and if your child breaks a rule, send him or her to timeout." I want to scream at these child behavioral specialists, "Our kids are different! This behavioral stuff just doesn't work for our kids. I am not a bad parent."

For years I had tried, with very limited success, to use a time out spot for my son for various bad behaviors, but I could never quite figure out why it didn't work the way the "behavioral specialists" said it would work. One day my son and daughter were playing in the back yard. They didn't really play; they mostly fought, and this day was no exception. I was standing near them, and my son picked up a stick and looked like he was planning to hit his sister with it. I quickly stepped in and using my most authoritative voice said, "Son, if you hit your sister with that stick, you will have to sit in timeout." There was a brief second when I could see him weighing the reward of getting to hit his sister with the consequence of sitting in timeout. He then turned quickly, hit her with the stick as hard as he could, and marched inside to sit in the timeout spot. I stared dumbfounded as he didn't look at me or say a word. I never used timeouts again! Our kids are different.

A timeout can be a great disciplinary tool for a lot of kids, but very seldom does it work for ours. There are two main drawbacks to timeouts for our kids. The first is that they simply don't see this as a punishment. In many cases, our children don't mind being in a quiet spot, away from the overly stimulating situations they were in before the timeout. Many times our kids can thrive on solitude and appreciate this being forced on them from time to time. It doesn't seem like much of a consequence, certainly not enough of a consequence to stop a bad behavior. Even in middle school, my son sometimes liked solitude. He would badger his only "mean" teacher mercilessly until she was angry enough that she gave him a silent lunch. He didn't really like sitting with all the other kids and talking to them while eating his lunch, so silent lunch was a nice break for him. The teacher never understood what was happening.

On the other spectrum, some children will simply refuse to go to timeout, and once parents resort to physical force to put the children into timeouts and keep them there, the benefits are lost. The children get huge amounts of attention. Most of our children don't care if the attention they get is negative or positive, as long as it is attention. So again, timeouts are not an effective consequence, and the bad behavior will usually continue.

The other discipline that typically does not work for our kids is spanking. Our kids have a very unique need for attention that is different than most kids. Our kids thrive on any kind of attention, which sounds odd since I just said that they typically don't mind sitting in timeout all by themselves. If I spank my child, he is getting negative attention. To him, negative attention is okay, and the bad behavior will continue. If I am angry while I am spanking him, he has an added bonus of feeling like he is controlling my emotions. So now he is getting attention and controlling my emotions, both things he loves.

Timeouts and spanking never worked for me. Following are some discipline techniques that I have found very useful. Every child is different, so of course I can't guarantee they will work. But if only half of them work, you will be well on your way to having a more peaceful and happy home.

Consequences and Rewards

Consequences and rewards are both ways to effectively discipline a child. I am a firm believer that every kid responds to these two discipline styles differently. It is important that all parents know which style is more effective for their children. I have one child that bristles if I even consider giving her a consequence, but she will rise to the occasion if I put a potential reward in front of her. The other child is just the opposite. If I put the best reward possible out there for him to attain, he will blow it every time. And on top of not receiving the reward, he will have a temper tantrum because he didn't get the reward, which he blames on me of course! He is much more compliant when I use consequences.

I once decided I would put the ultimate reward out there for him. We had two tickets to an NBA basketball game on Friday night. If he was able to come home from school three out of the five days in the week on green, which most kids in his class did every day anyway, he could go to the game with his father. Monday ended, and he came home unhappy because he was on red, not green. Tuesday ended, and he was dejected because again he came home on red, not green. We talked about what happened, but he squarely blamed the teacher for his inability to attain a status of green. The stress was building; he wanted to go to this game really badly. Once again, on Wednesday he came home on red and had a full-blown temper tantrum demanding that he get to go to the game anyway and that it wasn't his fault. The rest of the week was a disaster, full of tantrums and disappointment. I never again put a reward in front of him to try to earn. When I needed a behavior changed, I took away something or imposed a consequence, and the results were substantially better. Know your child and what they respond to best, a consequence or a reward.

Delayed Consequences

Some will say that dolling out an immediate consequence when a child commits an infraction is the only way to give consequences. The theory is that if you take immediate action, your child will more easily associate the consequence with the crime. This might be the case for younger children, but once they hit elementary school age, they are perfectly capable of remembering their crimes. Typically, if there is a temper tantrum or other problem, our children are upset and angry. This is the most inappropriate time to throw a consequence at them. In addition, we already have the consequence published as part of the list of rules. They know what the consequence will be because we have shared it with them.

The Love and Logic class we will talk about in the third part of this book (page 147) would handle a computer or "screen" problem like this: First, we already established the rule that there will be no screens if the child has a temper tantrum when asked to get off of the computer. When a child has the temper tantrum, Love and Logic would say, "Awww. I love you too much to fight with you. I will take care of this." And walk away. The child may not know the first few times you use this line that it means the consequence will be given later, but they will catch on quickly. The idea is to then administer the consequence the next time.

Here is a good example. My son will sometimes have a temper tantrum when I ask him to get off his computer and get ready for church. This is clearly on the list of rules, and he knows the consequence. When he throws a temper tantrum, I will say, "Awwww. I love you too much to fight about this. I will take care of this," and walk out of the room to finish getting ready. He will keep up his bad attitude, and I will ignore him the best I can. Next Sunday he comes downstairs, and the iPad is missing. He can't find the remote to the TV, and the power cord for the computer is gone. As he fumes and steams his way upstairs to complain, I calmly say, "Awwww. It is too bad that you don't have any screens before church this week. You had such a bad attitude last week, I thought this would help make it easier for you to get ready." Of course, this is where our kids will be furious and display their worst possible behavior.

Can you see who now has the upper hand? When I use this approach, I am not mad at all, and he cannot pull me into his misery. I know I have won. I made my point. If he doesn't get ready for church, the same thing will happen next Sunday. I can pretty easily ignore the temper tantrum this week and even a little name-calling. (Although I will make him write about it later. See "Removing Bad Words" in Week 8.)

Next Sunday, can you guess what happens? He has all his screens back, but the minute I say, "It is time to get ready for church," he immediately gets ready, without any attitude.

This type of discipline takes some planning and more time than screaming at our kids does, but it ends a lot of parental frustration and, in the end, more quickly gains compliance for basic family rules.

Discipline Is for the Next Time

One of the biggest mistakes we make as parents is hoping to gain compliance immediately for an infraction. We do this by screaming at our kids and hoping that they will magically shape up, right this minute. We set up ourselves for failure when we do this because everyone is in a heightened emotional state and not set up to learn anything right this minute. But if a situation is handled calmly, you can make sure the infraction doesn't happen again. Discipline is almost always for the next time a child does something, not for this time.

This makes most discipline an extreme inconvenience the first time you do what you say you are going to do. The lesson is the same for parents as it is for children. If you suffer through this the first time, you will be ultimately grateful that you don't have to suffer through it many, many more times in the future.

My husband and I happened to be driving separate cars and met at Chick-fil-A for dinner. Alex decided where he wanted the family to sit. That would have been fine, but he was being defiant and controlling about the seating arrangement, and we never give in to that kind of behavior. We sat at a different table and asked him to nicely come join us. He was close to a melt down, but I didn't say a word. I calmly but very firmly took his hand and headed to the car to avoid as much embarrassment as possible. I drove the 10 minutes home with Alex in the back seat wailing at the top of his lungs. When we got home, he calmed down a bit knowing he was not going back. We ate leftovers, and he went to bed. Nothing needed to be said. There was no screaming on my part. There were no lectures. He got the message loud and clear. There was never another defiant, controlling moment at Chick-fil-A or any other restaurant. It was worth the pain of the initial discipline to know in the future he would behave at restaurants. Every time he started to misbehave, we just said, "Remember the last time," and although we weren't always in a position to follow through like we had that evening, he was always much more compliant at restaurants.

Many times it is just not convenient to discipline kids, so we let them get away with it. There are times when the inconvenience is worth it. Find a few of those times and plan in advance how you will handle a temper tantrum if it happens. In the long run, it will be well worth the time and effort—and the embarrassment!

Consequences When They Are Sleeping

Another way to give consequences is when our little cherubs are sleeping. It is impossible to ask them to give us their screens, but it is easy to take them in the middle of the night. Computers can either be unplugged, or we used a computer app called TimesUpKidz that could be changed to disallow any screen time on certain days or at certain hours.

Alex was playing wildly in his chair and knocked it over. I told him calmly that if he knocked it over again, that night I would remove the chair for a week, and he could stand while using his computer. This worked really well. Previously I might have tried to take the chair away while he was there. This would have resulted in a physical matchup to see who could take the chair, and it would have gotten ugly. He didn't knock the chair over again, but if he had, it would have been easy for me to put the chair somewhere that night after he had gone to bed where he couldn't retrieve it. Say nothing about the missing chair the next day.

This worked the same way with his homework. His homework on Tuesdays was to write five very long, well-written sentences, as I mentioned earlier. We struggled through Tuesdays the best we could. Alex was determined not to do this homework. I would calmly say, "If you go out to play before your sentences are complete, while you are outside I will remove your computer. With a lot of drama, he finished his sentences and then only had 10 minutes to play outside, instead of an hour. The consequence was perfect. I wouldn't have actually removed his computer, but would have taken the power cord, which is much easier than hiding an entire computer! The next week, his sentences were done with much less drama, and everyone was happier.

Defer the Question

If you don't have an immediate answer to a demanding question, it is perfectly okay not to answer their question. Defer it until later. A good example of this is the classic dessert question. You sit down in a restaurant, and the first thing your child asks is if he can have dessert. If you say no, you are in for a full-blown tantrum, and you haven't even ordered yet. If you don't say anything, he will keep asking over and over again. If you say yes, he won't eat dinner but will save his appetite for the dessert you promised him. This is a lose-lose deal. The way to handle this is to defer the question. In your most pleasant tone say, "I don't know if you can have dessert because you haven't eaten your meal yet. Please ask me after you finish eating and if you ask before that the answer will be no." Then quickly redirect your child to something else, like coloring one of those kids menus or playing tic-tac-toe! That doesn't commit you to anything. After the meal, when your child again asks about dessert, you can still say yes or no, but now you are in a better place to head out the door if you say no and a tantrum ensues. This can also work in a grocery store when your child asks for candy, cookies, and so forth. You might choose to reward your child for good behavior in the store, but you won't know that until you are in the checkout line. Or if you are planning on saying no, you won't know until you have already checked out (you can only pull this one off with small children who don't quite understand the buying process yet).

I committed the sin of "yes" just last week. My child wanted to make the night special and pick out a movie to watch. I had a few extra minutes, so at 5:30 p.m., right before dinner, I helped him pick out a movie and said we could sit down and watch it after dinner. However, after dinner, he wanted to go out and play kickball, and then we got caught up in other outdoor activities. All of a sudden it was 8 p.m. and bedtime, and—you guessed it—he was ready to watch the movie I said yes to earlier! A full-blown tantrum ensued. In retrospect, I could have still picked out the movie when I did, but not said yes to watch it after dinner. We could have put the movie in a special place, and I could have said, "Next time we watch a movie, this is what we will watch. Wait until after dinner to ask me if we can watch it tonight."

Set Expectations

I can't say this often enough: our kids are so demanding that we have to set expectations a lot more frequently than most parents, and sometimes we are just too tired or distracted to be up for the task. When this happens, defer the question and then stop and decide what you want the expectation to be because the question will come back up all too soon. Here are a few examples. My son and I loved to go to a theme park during the summer. He would ask me repeatedly for a piece of candy. It made the whole day a disaster for me, and I was so frustrated by the end of the day that I swore I would never return. I gave some thought to what I was okay giving him while at the park, and the next time we went, this is what I said: "Son, I am fine with you getting one piece of candy or one sweet thing, such as ice cream while we are at the park. And you can pick anything you want as long as it does not cost more than $5. But you are not allowed to have it until just before we leave for the day." I gave him control over what he chose for his sweet item, and I gave him at least a little control over when he could have it. We headed to the park. Within 30 minutes, he asked for candy. I calmly replied, "Sure you can have candy. So are you ready to leave already?" I had to remind him of the new rule at least four or five times before he got it. At the end of the day, we spent 30 minutes picking out the candy, and he chose a huge multi-colored lollipop. Not my favorite due to all the chemical dyes in it, but I was going to keep my word no matter what he chose. It was a fabulous day! From then on, when we went to the theme park, he would only ask once or twice for something before he realized that I was going to stick to this rule. Just a side note here—theme parks or large noisy places are very tough for our kids to handle, can cause sensory overload and out of control behavior. If at all possible, opt for a season pass, and then if your child seems to be at the end of his rope half way through the day, get him his treat and call it a day. Don't push to the point of a full-blown tantrum while walking out of the park. I am sure I don't need to tell you how embarrassing those are!

Summer is pool season, and our pool happens to have a snack bar. Some kids get unlimited use of the snack bar, but if I did that for my kid, he would eat his dinner in junk food from the snack bar every day. Decide what you will be comfortable giving. Is it one ice cream or candy a day? Is it a dollar each day? Is it a dollar a week? If at all possible, the answer shouldn't just be no. Try to compromise a little bit and give your children some control. Let's say the comfortable thing is a snack once a week, but it has to be something without dyes in it, such as chocolate. So tell him they are allowed one snack at the snack bar per week. Let him decide which day of the week that will be, and then make a big deal out of the great decision he makes. The more buy in you get from your children, the less hassle when it really happens. You can also let your children decide if they want the money to purchase what they want or if they want you to do this for them (if you are okay with this). Together you can decide what items they like the best. You get the idea here. Try to give them control over as many things as possible. The feeling of control calms our kids down. It stops them from bristling all the time and waiting for our next decree to come down from on high.

Technology and Consequences

I could fill a whole book with ideas related to technology and our kids, but let me start with just a few observations. Most of our kids love their devices. I call them screens, which includes anything that has a screen such as the TV, iPhone, iTouch, iPad, Xbox—you get the idea. Our kids love screens because they are predictable. They can get an endorphin rush from winning and moving to the next level. If they lose, they get to try again until they do win, and no one ever lectures them.

Parents constantly ask me how much screen time their children should have. A good rule of thumb is children not yet in kindergarten shouldn't have more than 30 minutes each day, and the screen time should be educational in nature. Once a child is in elementary school, 30 minutes of any screen is still enough but doesn't need to be as educational—think Minecraft, Clash of Clans, and so forth. By middle school, one to two hours is plenty, and half of that time should be TV time and not interactive computer time, especially as it gets closer to bedtime.

Screens of any kind, including television should never be in a child's room. This is a sure way for a child to get into a great deal of trouble, some of which could compromise safety as he or she gets older.

The main reason I finally gave in and purchased an iPhone for my son was so that I could take it away from him. Any type of screen seems to be a great consequence for disciplinary actions.

I highly recommend that at a very young age, you put some rules around screen time. One of my favorites is to require exercise immediately after the children are done with their screen time. Children get mean when they are on their screens, and exercise makes them nice again. This might sound funny but it is true of most kids. A good exercise that can be done regardless of the weather outside is jumping on a mini trampoline. Kids love to do this, and if it gets boring, you can spice it up by throwing a ball to them while they are jumping. Have them jump small and large jumps in a sequence. Have them jump really high or really low. There are all sorts of variations. Of course, if it's a nice day outside, running around the house or any number of other activities will work just as well.

Tantrums

Our kids have tantrums and more tantrums and more tantrums. It seems like a release for them, and the more they can draw you into the battle the better. That makes them feel powerful. Tantrums in our kids are not always about getting things they want. They happen because our children are almost always out of control or right on the brink, and the slightest little things will push them over the edge. A tantrum releases those feelings of frustration. When adults are sad or anxious, we often have lots of pent-up emotions, so sometimes we cry to release those emotions. When our kids are out of control or angry, they have tantrums to release those emotions. At first glance, tantrums seem to be about getting something they want, but more often than not, they are just about releasing those emotions that have built up over the last few seconds or minutes due to frustrating situations. If you are at home, walking out of the room is a great strategy, although you might have to find a good hiding spot so that they don't follow you around the house screaming. A temper tantrum without an audience doesn't accomplish its intended results.

Walk Away

My son can be very demanding: "Mom! Mom! Mom! Get me the milk. Get me a spoon. Get me this. Get me that." I think I have already iterated that I am not my child's maid or his butler, and I seldom get him the things he is asking for, especially if he asks me in a rude, disrespectful way. But our kids are different than other kids; they will keep asking. They don't care if the answer is no; they just like asking, maybe hoping to get a negative emotion, which they can feed off of. Just walk away. When my son is in the kitchen eating his cereal and starts that line of demands, I simply walk outside and shut the door, or walk upstairs or go get the newspaper. I don't even answer him. That might seem rude, but if I give him any answer, to him that is an open invitation to start a fight or have a temper tantrum. Here is one of the most important rules you can learn: your child can't act out if he or she is the only one in the room!

CHAPTER 16

Week 6: Chores and Allowance

Chores are a constant struggle for our kids. They don't get the concept of helping around the house and assume that this is the parents' job. Nothing makes me more furious than an eight year old asking me to do something, and when I say no he says, "But, Mom, you don't do anything. Why can't you do this for me?" I don't think this is insolence. I think kids really don't have any idea how many jobs parents have to do.

Let's change this. Put a large notebook on the counter or tape a very large sheet of paper to the refrigerator. Ask everyone in the house to write down all the things they do to contribute to the household. Leave the list for a couple of weeks, and as you or the kids think of other things, add to the list. If a parent adds an item such as "go to work to make money for the family," it is fair for the child to write "go to school to learn." Don't put any names next to the items as you write them. We are going to do this later.

Wash dishes	Mow lawn	Sweep steps
Vacuum	Clean bathroom sinks	Clean toilets
Go to school	Clean litter box	Fix toilets
Do homework	Feed dog	Wash dog
Wash car	Mop kitchen floor	Go to work
Grocery shopping	Clean kitchen sink	Pack lunch
Make dinner	Clean up after dinner	Unload dishwasher

Now it's time to call a family meeting to review the list. The idea is to assign each of these items to a person in the household so that the list is somewhat fair. When this is complete, the list might look something like this.

Alex	Heather
Clean Bathroom Sinks	Mop Kitchen Floors
Sweep Steps	Wash Dishes
Mow Lawn	Feed Dog
Pack Lunch	Pack Lunch
Go To School	Go To School
Do Homework	Do Homework
Mom	**Dad**
Grocery Shopping	Vacuum
Make Dinner	Fix Toilets
Clean Toilets	Wash Cars
Unload Dishwasher	Clean Up After Dinner
Wash Dog	Go To Work

There should be about the same number of items for each family member, suggesting that everyone helps out and everyone does his or her fair share of the general household duties. Even if you have much younger children that can't do as much, add things to their lists such as empty trash cans, set the table, fill the dog's water bowl, or other responsibilities that the children are able to accomplish on their own.

Now that all items have been assigned, it is a good idea to record the children's contributions. A white board or list pinned to the wall is a good way to designate the contributions made by each child and when they should be done. This way, the parent can refer to the list or the whiteboard instead of to individual contributions. "Have you completed everything on the whiteboard?" is a much better inquiry than, "Have you cleaned your room, emptied the trash, and mopped the floors?" The second question, when compared to the first question, will more likely lead to a confrontation.

After you have determined what your child will do to help out the family, add the timing to the board or list. List the completion time instead of the start time. When my children have weekend contributions, I list the end time as 9 p.m. Sunday evening. This usually means the items get done at 8 p.m. Sunday evening, but that is okay as long as they don't roll into the next week. This also assumes that I will not be nagging them all weekend. As a parent, I must be able to control my need to control them. If I am unable to do this, then I need to change the end time to something in the middle of the weekend, such as Saturday at 5 p.m.

If you had a job assignment that was due Friday by 5 p.m., your boss would not nag you all week to get it done. In fact, your boss would likely not care if you pulled an all-nighter on Thursday night to complete the project. As long as it was successfully completed by the agreed upon time, everyone would be happy.

Our children are capable of so much more than we give them credit. They are constantly fighting for control, so giving them control over little things like the timing of when they do their contributions is easy. Of course, there does have to be a consequence for not completing the task at the agreed upon time.

The white board might look something like this.

Contribution	When	Consequence if not completed
Dog – food and water	Morning before school	I let my child think that the dog will be hungry all day
Clean litter box	Before dinner daily	No dinner until clean
Mop kitchen floors	Weekend before 5 p.m. Sunday	No iPhone until Monday afternoon and task is complete
Laundry	When clothes are dirty	Wear dirty clothes
Empty trash	When mom says	Must complete one of parents chores
Take trash cans to the curb	Monday night by 8 p.m.	Parent will wake you in middle of night to complete task
Put dirty dishes in dishwasher	After dinner before leaving the kitchen	Parent will remind you at an inconvenient time to do this
Unload the dishwasher	When parent says they are clean	Must complete one of parents' chores

Have a few daily tasks as well as a few weekend tasks. If there are tasks such as mowing the lawn, those will likely need a gentle reminder since most lawns do not need to be mowed at exactly the same time each week or month. You can't expect a child to notice when the grass needs to be mowed. Typically, even your husband needs a gentle reminder to do certain tasks, so don't think your kids are super human. Gentle reminders and nagging multiple times are entirely different. After you have reminded a child once and you are sure he or she has heard you (you have gotten some type of response), there should be no more reminders. The consequence will occur.

Contributions to the family should start at a very young age. A child as young as four or five is capable of setting the table. Here are some age-appropriate contributions to the household.

Child's Age	Contribution
3–5	Set the table Clean their room or playroom (with your help) Match and put away socks and underwear
6–10	Laundry Help Pack School Lunch Clean Sinks Empty Trash Cans Sweep porch or walkway
11–14	Take Trash to/from curb Clean entire bathroom Mop Floors Load/Unload Dishwasher
15+	Mow Lawn Plan and cook one meal every week

Many parents will give their children an allowance for doing their chores. Since chores have been renamed to family contributions, should the child get paid for these? Do parents get paid for doing their family contributions? No.

I believe children should be given some money on a regular basis in order to learn how to spend and save. I have moved to a monthly allowance because I could not remember to give the money to my kids every week. Things got confrontational when I couldn't remember whether I had paid allowance and the child was sure I had not. When I pay monthly allowance, I write a little note on my calendar so that there is never any doubt whether it was paid or not. I have also changed the name of allowance to "practice money." It is their money to practice spending and saving while in a nurturing environment. If they don't get a chance to do this with a few dollars when they are young, they could run into some very bad consequences when they are adults.

The amount of practice money should be in direct proportion to how many things the child is responsible for purchasing. At a very young age, the child might not be responsible for purchasing anything, but as they get older, they might have to spend their money to purchase gifts for others, especially at Christmas. They might have to pay for any snacks or extras when they are at a restaurant or movie. I have a few friends who will give their teenagers $100 per month, and they have to purchase everything they need, from schoolbooks to clothes to movie tickets to being on a sports team. This really gets them thinking about money management when they want to purchase that $150 pair of Nike sneakers. Each child has different needs so each should have a different allowance and be responsible for different things if they are different ages.

Fair and Even Are Different

I have two children. There are 28 children in each child's school classroom. Some would say that all children should be treated the same. If one gets to write on the chalkboard, they should all have a turn. Each kid should have a chance to answer a question before being called on a second time. That is an equal way to look at things, but it is not fair.

I always tell my children that equal and fair are two completely different things. In other words, things don't always have to be equal to be fair. My children are different, so my parenting has to be different. They can't compare themselves to their siblings, and they can't compare how I parent one child to how I parent the other child.

I would argue that if everything is even between children, it is not fair. Treating children fairly takes into account their differences and their individual needs. My children have different bedtimes because they need different amounts of sleep. One of my children has harder chores than the other because that one is more capable of completing those chores.

It is perfectly acceptable for a parent to make those choices. Don't let your kids decide that everything should be even. Each child has his or her own privileges based on merits. Period.

CHAPTER 17

Week 7: Control, Praise and Attention

Choices and Control

Our kids are control freaks. I think I have already said this. The younger they are, the worse problems this creates. It is hard to give a four-year-old a lot of control. They can't make their own food. They can't give themselves a bath. They can't make household decisions. They don't have the mental or physical capacity to be in control. Even though all these things are true, our kids need to be in control. There were times when I could see Alex noticeably calm down when he perceived that he was in control of a situation.

In order to give younger children the feeling of control, we need to give them lots of choices. They should have at least a half dozen choices each day that they perceive as important. Here are the basic rules for choices.

- Give a child two choices—never more than that.
- Either choice should be okay with the parent.
- If they don't choose within five seconds, choose for them and do not discuss the choice again. Move on.

Here are some examples:

- Would you like rice or mashed potatoes with dinner tonight?
- Would you like to use the oatmeal or lemon soap next?
- Would you like a cookie or a piece of candy for dessert?
- Would you like to buy regular or chocolate milk for lunch?
- Do you want to throw a football or baseball around?

The nice thing about control is as children grow up, they can continue to take on more responsibilities and be a larger part of family decision-making, which appeases their intense desire to control everything.

If your child fights to make his or her own decisions, consider giving up some of the things you do for him or her. At the age of nine, my son started doing his own laundry. At 11 he started packing his own lunch for school each day (staying within preset parameters). The more control I gave him, the better a kid he became. And the more things for which he took responsibility and did well, the more I was able to praise his good choices.

Alex continually asked me to say yes more often. He would try to bargain with me. "If you say yes more often, I will be a better kid and do what you ask me to do." By the time Alex was a rising fifth grader, he was 10 years old and was able to stay at the neighborhood pool without my supervision. I was not really comfortable with that, but I knew he would be safe because there were multiple lifeguards and he was a good swimmer. I told him I would let him go to the pool whenever he wanted to go, assuming it wasn't a major inconvenience to me. He could call me on the phone when he wanted to come home, and in return, he would say yes to my requests more often. Knowing this would fail miserably, I sent him to the pool and even gave him $5 to purchase lunch or whatever he wanted. I didn't tell him not to purchase candy or sodas or give him any instructions. I told him I was excited that he was now old enough to make his own decisions and trusted he would make good ones. By the end of the week, I was amazed at the transformation in my child. He came home one day bragging about the good lunch he purchased with his $5.

The trust I showed in him came back to me a hundred fold. He was calmer and an easier kid to be around that entire summer. As Alex calmed down, I calmed down, and the whole family seemed calmer.

I was also able to teach lessons when the choices weren't as good. Some choices had their own built-in consequences, like the time Alex didn't pull his favorite white shirt out of the dark load of laundry, and it ended up a light shade of pink. There was no need for a lecture. He never made that mistake again. It was a great lesson to learn with a cheap white shirt, instead of learning the lesson at an older age with an expensive designer shirt. So bring on the mistakes at an early age!

Mistakes Please

Children seem so vulnerable when they are young. As moms, we have a deep, almost uncontrollable need to protect them from the harsh, cruel world they face every day. One of the hardest things to do is to get out of our kids' way and let them make mistakes. Making mistakes, as a child or as an adult, is one of the best ways to learn new things. We cripple our kids when we don't let them make mistakes, and then they don't learn valuable life lessons. The consequence when a five year old takes something from a store is not severe, relatively speaking. He takes something from the store, his mother discovers it, and she marches him back to face the manager and admit his crime. He is ashamed and knows he has let down his parents. There is a good probability that he will never take anything again. The opposite scenario is the mother who watches her children like a hawk and keeps them from taking anything. Those children don't learn the very valuable lesson about not taking things that are not theirs. At age 18, if they take something that doesn't belong to them, the consequence might be jail time.

Pray for your children to make lots of mistakes when they are young. The consequences are much more lenient, and the lessons learned are invaluable. As long as the mistake doesn't cause any bodily harm or hurt another person, we should try to help our children make as many mistakes as possible.

School is another place where parents tend to want to help but end up getting in the way. Elementary school is the perfect time to learn what happens when you don't turn in homework. Usually the child has to walk some extra laps at recess or do his homework in class while the other children are doing a fun activity. School is fully equipped to handle that issue, and I want it handled in elementary school, not in high school where the stakes are higher.

I do understand that sometimes even moms forget things and need someone to bail them out. If my children forget their homework or their lunch, I typically will take a lunch or homework to school as long as it doesn't become a habit. We then talk about how to keep from forgetting things. Ideas include packing the night before, going through a mental checklist in your head before walking out the door, and putting your school things in a certain place every day. This is a great learning experience.

As we let our children make mistakes they can learn from, it is important to step in if there is a decision that could hurt a child or create a long-term setback. In one of our parenting classes, there was a 15-year-old who wanted to be on the dive team but wasn't interested in getting the paperwork filled out. As a parent, I would step in and fill out the paperwork for him. He would learn a lesson if he didn't fill out the paperwork and couldn't participate in the dive team. On the other hand, there is such a huge benefit to being on a team, competing against others, improving on a skill you enjoy, that the benefit to stepping in and helping outweighs the costs. There will be other times to learn a lesson with less of an overall impact on the child's life.

A Pat on the Back

A chapter on discipline would not be complete without talking about positive behavior. Sometimes we get so caught up in our children's negative behavior that we forget to tell them if they do a good job. I read an article that said ADHD children hear 20,000 more negative comments than other children.

Our kids seldom get pats on the back at school or when playing on athletic teams or any place else. They are usually getting discipline notes to send home!

Someone has to tell them they are doing a good job. If you haven't found a time during the day to tell them what they did right, be sure to tell them when you are putting them to bed. Don't lecture. Just make it a passing comment—something like, "You did a great job finishing your homework today. I was proud of you," "thanks for eating all your dinner tonight," or "I am glad you didn't fight with your sister today. You are really growing up."

Just one sentence once a day is enough to get your point across. Your children may not even acknowledge what you said, but they did hear you. After you give your compliment, continue on with what you were doing without saying anything else about it.

This may sound like a small and insignificant piece of advice, but it is very important. You are changing how you discipline, and you have stopped yelling, so now it is time for a little well-deserved praise!

CHAPTER 18

Week 8: Other Ideas

Removing Bad Words from a Child's Vocabulary

Many of you may not deem this a priority, but the words listed below were being used way too often in our house. The disrespect needed to stop, so we implemented the following approach. This has been one of the easiest things for our family to fix.

Let's use one of the things that our children are typically not very good at—their writing skills. Even if you have a child who writes well, this will probably work. Here is the setup. Sit down with all the children in the house and tell them that certain words are no longer going to be used—ever. Give them a list of words that you want removed from their vocabulary, or ask for their help to come up with the list. My list looked like this:

- Shut up
- Stupid
- Idiot
- God (when swearing)
- Liar (when talking to parents)

Bring out a notebook and set it next to the list. When any of these words are spoken, the offender must write 10 times in the book that they will not use this word again. There will be no (insert consequence here), until this has been done. Meeting adjourned. Don't get into any negotiation or any discussion on this new rule; just leave the room and if necessary the house. Walk outside to check on the mail or to pull a couple of weeds in the yard. You must end the conversation and not get into any battle over this new rule.

Be sure you know exactly what the consequence is going to be, and be prepared to stick to it. I usually use something that is going to happen soon, like a meal: "you cannot eat dinner until you have written your 10 sentences;" or "you cannot have computer time until you have written your 10 sentences;" or "I have a brownie here for your dessert, but you can't have it until you finish those sentences." Don't use a consequence where you take away something. Just defer something they want to do until the sentences are written.

Do not give any second chances on this rule. When the first infraction occurs, calmly get the notebook, write the sentence once: "I will not tell my sister to shut up." Or "I will never call an adult a liar." Or "I will never call my friend an idiot." Number the page one through 10, give the notebook to your child, reiterate the consequence, and walk out of the room as fast as possible. Stay as far away from the "crime scene" as possible but close enough to be able to administer the consequence if necessary. In other words, you don't want your child to throw the notebook across the room and get onto the computer when you are not paying attention. At the same time, you want to be as far away as possible when your child throws a tantrum about this new rule. Remember that a tantrum is not nearly as effective if you aren't there to hear it! When your child complies, let him or her have whatever you were withholding without another word and without a lecture. If the 10 sentences are illegible, don't say a word and don't make him or her do it again. You have made your point. Don't rub it in! My son has even written "I WILL tell my sister to shut up" 10 times! That is his little way of saving face in a bad situation. I have still made my point. The lesson has been learned. I gave him what I was withholding as the consequence and moved on.

Here is what the sheet might look like:

I will not tell my sister to shut up

1.

2.

3.

4.

5.

6.

7.

8.

9.

10.

I have found that it doesn't take long with this method to clean up their vocabulary. Most ADHD kids hate to write, and this is a situation when I think it is okay to play on that weakness!

I have to pull out this discipline about once a year as my children start to add bad words back to their vocabulary. It is much easier to do each subsequent time it is needed. Now, I usually pull out the notebook and put it on the table, and the bad words and name-calling stop.

Car Behavior

I am sure everyone has endured bickering between kids and all-out fights in the car while mom is trying very hard to concentrate on driving and getting to the destination safely. Here is a fun trick that worked for me. The results will depend on your kids' personality types. My son insisted on starting an argument, having a temper tantrum, or throwing stuff in the car. He was bored and refused to pack anything to do while driving. I refused to let him take screens in the car because when we got to our destination, there was always a five-minute delay while he finished playing his game, which drove me through the roof. So I put a magazine in the car and asked my older child to do the same thing. The next time the boy child even started to fuss, I found a safe neighborhood to park. I calmly pulled out my magazine and stated, "It has become unsafe for me to drive while you are arguing with your sister. When you are done, we can keep driving." Of course, the tantrum persisted, but I sat and read my magazine. Sometimes I had to get out of the car and read my magazine outside to avoid the screams. Eventually everything calmed down, and we continued on our journey. Now, don't think this will work immediately to solve all bickering in the car. I had to do this at least a dozen times before I got some peace and quiet in the car. In the end, my son decided to put a *Guinness Book of World Records* in the car, and when I pulled over to read, he got out his book to read. As long as everyone was reading or at least looking at the pictures, it became "safe" for me to drive again. This suggestion does take some planning. Since my child had a tantrum almost every time we got in a car, I could pick specific trips to leave 15 minutes early, knowing I would be sitting in a neighborhood reading a magazine while a temper tantrum subsided. I have had calm, mostly uneventful car rides for many years now, after investing about 10 trips using this method. Our kids are tenacious and will not take to this quickly, especially if they have spent years making car rides miserable. Most disciplines involve the parent being inconvenienced first before the child learns the lesson. Just keep telling yourself that a quiet car for years to come is worth investing in now.

I have a friend who plans an immediate retreat on the first trip to the pool in the summertime. Inevitably, her children will start bickering in the car. She simply turns the car around and goes home. She has already planned for this and tells me that it happens like clockwork every year. All discipline is easier if you are prepared for it. If they ever surprise you and don't start bickering, then you can enjoy that day at the pool and maybe even treat them to an ice cream for their good car behavior.

Calendar on the Wall

This isn't so much a discipline technique as a good way for everyone in the family to know what is going on from day to day. I have tried electronic versions of the calendar, but unless your children are all old enough to have an electronic calendaring system, the old-fashioned way has worked best for me. I have a large wall calendar with three different colored markers: purple for my daughter, red for my son, and black for the parents. Everything goes on the calendar. Each day, the children can look at the calendar and see what they are doing or what the family is doing.

Since I am making appointments when I am not at home staring at the wall calendar, I take a picture of the calendar every few weeks and mark it as a favorite on my phone. I now have my own electronic calendar to reference. I put new appointments in my phone as notes and transfer them to my wall calendar every few days.

There are many ways to tackle calendars. As long as your children can visually see what is happening in their world and what the rest of the family is doing, use whatever method works best for your family.

Here is an example of our wall calendar:

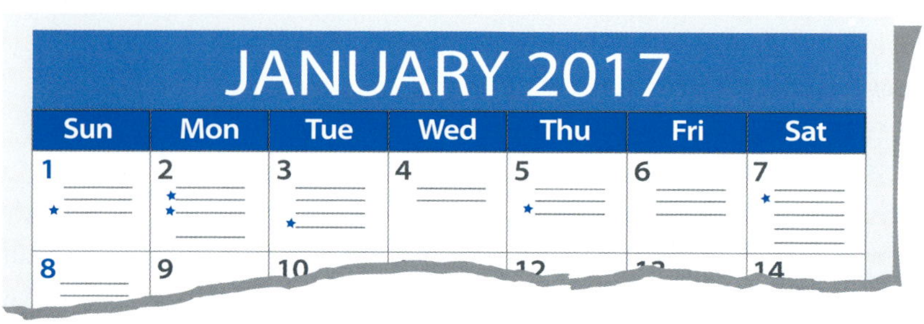

Happy Birthday!

Don't ever miss a birthday to give more responsibilities to a child. I will sometimes even purchase a cake and celebrate half birthdays just because it is a great excuse to change up some of the chores and give more responsibilities because they are now "older" and much more capable of handling additional responsibilities. Our kids *can* handle lots of things, but they just don't *want* to handle them. It's really important to sell them on the idea and get buy in from them, and a birthday is the perfect time to do it. Keep in mind that our children thrive as we continue to give them control of their lives. This includes helping around the house.

Additional Tips

Here are a few extra tips when administering discipline.

1) Sit when disciplining. That means you, not the child! Hovering over a child is a bad way to administer discipline. I have found that one of the best ways to talk to a child is while walking the dog. That way you are not looking directly at each other, and the child is more likely to open up and talk to you. I call it a walk and talk. If you don't have a dog, try throwing a ball around or kicking a soccer ball back and forth.
2) When your child does something wrong, consider starting your inquisition out with something less demanding, like "I'm curious why you didn't call when you said you would." This can open up a discussion without causing them to shut down immediately. Another good opener is "that doesn't sound like you—can you tell me what happened?"
3) Our kids can get hyper focused on something of interest to them. Look for hobbies and things to do that play to this personality trait. For some, it might be Legos or other building blocks. For others, it might be making something artistic.

Summary

If you were able to follow the elimination diet and discover food sensitivities in your child, you did an awesome job! In addition, you may have added supplements your child was lacking or removed toxins that produced a bad reaction. If your child has been misbehaving in a certain way for years and is used to certain behaviors, this section has likely helped. If there are any remaining symptoms, the next section lists additional interventions that can be implemented.

PART THREE:

Interventions

CHAPTER 19

Celebrate Calm

This is the first intervention I want to discuss, although from a chronological standpoint, we didn't come across this strategy until Alex was eight. This is the one intervention that probably saved our child and changed our lives. That's a pretty strong statement, but it is 100 percent true.

From the day Alex entered the United States, he was a strong-willed, fussy, unhappy child. I would go as far as saying he was angry and mean-spirited most of the time. As parents, we felt like we saved his life by adopting him and removing him from deplorable conditions. A little gratitude every once in awhile might have been nice. Kids just don't see things the same way as adults, and no matter how many lectures we gave on being grateful or being respectful, my son was still ungrateful and disrespectful. I am sure everyone has heard the common adage "insanity is doing the same thing over and over again and expecting different results." Why, as parents, do we yell and scream the same things over and over again and expect different results? Insanity? I doubt it! The reasons are simple:

- We don't know what else to do.
- We want to win the argument.
- We want to teach our children the right things.
- We are too tired to do anything else!

If we were honest with ourselves, we would realize that we don't win the arguments and rarely teach our children the right things when we are having our own temper tantrums. We haven't accomplished our parenting objectives.

Our kids know exactly which buttons to push to make us mad. Our kids also want to win the argument, and they are control freaks. If they can't get their way or get us to buy them something they want, then the consolation prize is to control our emotions and make us mad.

Every time they make us frustrated, angry, or mad and we give them visible signs that our emotions are out of control, they have won. This is what

I never understood when I had out-of-control arguments with Alex.

At the tender age of three, he would ask for crazy things that he knew he wouldn't get or wouldn't happen. I have already told part of this story once, but I am going to tell it again. Almost every day we drove to school and he would demand that I turn left at a certain stop light. He knew school was to the right. I turned right, and he would scream and have a temper tantrum. That would set me off, and pretty soon we would both be screaming at each other the rest of the way to school. He won. He was in total control of my emotions. He got to school and was happy that he won. I kissed him, and he toddled off to play. I was a wreck!

One day I was desperately searching the Internet for some type of intervention that could help. I found a set of CDs called *Celebrate Calm* by Kirk Martin. They were expensive, but when compared to counseling or most of the other interventions I researched, they were not really expensive at all. I ordered the CDs and as soon as they arrived sat down to listen to the first one. All those times I allowed arguments to escalate so that I could "win" the argument, I had lost. My child wanted those arguments to escalate because he feeds on the negative emotions and wins. In the end, even if I made my point and I never gave into what he was asking, I still lost because he got what he wanted—my negative emotions that he thought he controlled.

This is where most parenting advice does not apply to our strong-willed children. I always thought that since I never gave in to him, I was doing the right thing. It never occurred to me that what he wanted, more than what he was demanding on that particular day, was to control my emotions. He was a master at it, and I was angry and frustrated.

I was not going to continue to allow my child to win, so I stopped yelling. I stopped losing. The *Celebrate Calm* CDs were the ultimate intervention, but after both my husband and I started using this approach, Alex's behavior escalated. At first, Alex was frustrated that he could no longer make us have negative emotions that he could feed off of. When we stopped screaming and stopped letting him win, he tried harder to make us mad. He tried harder to make us scream. He didn't know what to do because he suddenly couldn't win an argument. We refused to yell anymore. He was mad, then very angry, and then furious. His behavior continued to escalate as if he was addicted to the screaming. He had to have it, and the only way he knew to get it was to do worse and worse things.

Our household began to escalate into violence at the hands of an eight-year-old child. There was no longer any yelling from us. When we asked Alex to do anything, he would try to hit me, grab my arms and twist them, or grab my hands and try to twist back my thumbs to hurt me. He perceived me as the weaker of the two parents. I always wanted my husband to be there when I was with Alex because I didn't want to be alone with him.

It was a scary time. It was a heart-breaking time. I researched homes that would take a violent child in if it came down to that. I knew that the minute my child grabbed a knife, he would no longer be able to live in our house again.

After asking around, my husband and I found a noted psychiatrist and had Alex evaluated. The psychiatrist equated my son's behavior to how a rat in a maze would act. If you give a rat food in the same place every day, he will go to that place every day. When the food is removed, he will continue to go to that place every day. He might rattle the cage or try other ways to get the food to appear, like it always has in the past. He would appear frustrated and noticeably irritated. After a period of time, he may only go to that place every other day, then once a week, and so forth until he finally forgets that food was ever in that place. Our children will respond the same way when we take something very important away from them—our negative emotions. The psychiatrist assured us that patience was the key. Teaching a child something that he needs to know should never involve arguing, anger, or outward frustration toward the child. It instead involves empathy and calm. This is one of the most important lessons I have learned, and it was not easy.

We had the most miserable six months of our lives after we started "calm parenting." Then, our lives and our family changed. Everything started getting better. We worked on smarter ways to get our point across, many of which are included in the eight-week discipline section. Sometimes we were rewarded with a calmer, happier child who started to internalize what we were trying to teach.

Sometimes this is one of the hardest lessons to apply on a daily basis. We are busy moms. We can be tired, frustrated, and angry, and we are human. There are times, though not often, that I still yell at my kids, and I immediately recognize that I need a time out, which is to say that I need to take care of myself a little more and stop spending so much time taking care of everyone else.

Visit celebratecalm.com to learn more.

> "I love you too much to fight with you. I will take care of this."
>
> Charles Fay, PhD, Love and Logic

CHAPTER 20

Love and Logic

Many times our children are out of control. We can medicate them to calm them down or to stimulate their brains, but we can also address some of the behaviors with certain disciplines that have been proven effective for our type of children. As your new diet begins to help calm your child, it is now important to eliminate some of those bad habits that have hung around for too long!

Love and Logic is one of these discipline programs. Charles Fay, PhD, and Jim Fay created the program with help from Foster W. Cline, MD. It is similar to *Celebrate Calm* in many ways. It espouses the need to be calm around kids and to exhibit a complete lack of emotion when children are out of control. It teaches a certain method to handle situations. It goes something like this:

1) Show empathy when your child comes to you with a problem.

2) Ask the child how he or she plans to fix the problem.

3) If he or she doesn't know, offer suggestions.

4) Walk away and wish your child luck with the problem.

Engaging in power struggles with our children, or any child for that matter, will seldom elicit the response we are looking for. After yelling at a child to comply with a house rule, I can't imagine that child ever saying, "Oh, I am so sorry, Mom. I will go do that right now. Thanks for pointing out the error of my ways." It just doesn't happen. If you want support from an excellent parenting organization to help you stop yelling at your children and start parenting in a calm, more effective way, search out a Love and Logic class or lecture.

For more details on finding a program, visit loveandlogic.com.

Our kids are seldom auditory learners, and yet most public and private schools expect them to sit quietly and listen the better part of each school day.

CHAPTER 21

Schools

I would consider the school your child attends as its own type of intervention. Our kids tend to have a lot of anxiety, and school is one of the worst offenders. I have always wondered if all of our children were homeschooled, whether any of them would ever be diagnosed with ADHD.

Our kids are seldom auditory learners, and yet most public and private schools expect them to sit quietly and listen the better part of each school day. When we sit them in a rigid school environment where they must be quiet and must listen all day, we set them up for frustration and usually failure. As parents, we have very little control over the public school environment and many times don't have the resources to consider moving our children to a private school. However, if there is a way to find the resources and move to a different school that more effectively meets your child's needs, don't hesitate to do it. It might end up being one of the best interventions you can choose for your child.

Our kids are typically highly visual and kinesthetic, so try to find a school that teaches the curriculum in this manner. They are not auditory. That shouldn't be a surprise to anyone as all of us have asked our children something for the tenth time and been totally ignored. There is a distinct possibility that your child actually did not hear you any of those 10 times. So imagine what must happen when a teacher is talking to our children for six or more hours of auditory learning each day. And we wonder why they come home on red each day or why we get calls from teachers that our children are once again misbehaving. Maybe the diagnosis should simply be "visual, kinesthetic learner" instead of ADHD. We can't change our society when it comes to school, but it is becoming easier to make different school choices as charter schools are added to the public school system and private schools that specialize in meeting our kid's needs, continue to grow and thrive. Some charter schools can be smaller and may specialize in something your child is interested in, such as math or science, while still being part of the public school system.

Montessori schools are typically a good fit for our children, although they can be expensive. Wikipedia describes Montessori education as "an educational approach developed by Italian physician and educator Maria Montessori based on her extensive research with 'phrenasthenic' or 'special needs' children and characterized by an emphasis on independence, freedom within limits, and respect for a child's natural psychological, physical, and social development." Montessori believed that children who are allowed to choose activities within an environment prepared according to her model would be well adjusted and open to educational challenges for optimal development.

There are typically mixed-age classrooms in a Montessori environment, which allows children with similar developmental needs to be grouped together. Many times there are choices of activities and a block of time, such as two to three hours, for the child to complete the activity with freedom of movement throughout the classroom. This gives our children a chance for control and autonomy without the rigorous structure of the public school system while still learning a complete curriculum designed for their developmental ages.

In many cities, there are also small schools with limited enrollment and high teacher-to-child ratios. If you are looking for an alternative to public schools, also consider start-up schools. They can cost less and still provide a great education. Although you may need to do more research, a school with only a few kids can give your child the break he or she needs from the high stress of public schools. I sent my daughter to one of these schools after she completed elementary school in the public school system. By fifth grade, we had her on 10 mg of Focalin. Her spirit was almost broken because she thought she was the dumbest child in the class, and she was starting to retreat inside herself. The only award she ever won was for perseverance, but that trait could only take her so far before it was also lost in the downward spiral of ADD. In her sixth grade year, I pulled her out of the public schools and sent her to a school that was just opening for its first year of instruction. She went to school that year with one teacher and two other boys. I don't think the curriculum was as strong as the public school, but the up side was that she learned all of it. In public school she might have learned 20 percent of the curriculum at best, due to the auditory way the curriculum is taught. I also stopped giving her medication. She was far better off in this small start up in the long run. After one year of this school, I moved her to a school that had about 30 children in each grade, six to eight children in a classroom with a teacher, and a stronger overall curriculum. She still didn't need any ADD medication. If her mind wandered, the teacher could always get her reengaged due to the small class size. She started coming home with straight As, her confidence returned, and she thrived in that environment. She turned into a smart, beautiful, amazing child, with the only intervention being a change of schools and, as she moved into high school, a cup of coffee to focus her for morning classes.

If you are stuck trying to make a public school work for your child, you most likely will need to setup a 504 plan or an IEP. I am not going to go into the details of these plans; plenty of information is available in books and on the Internet on how to set one up.

If you find a school you think might be a good fit, be sure to present this option in a low key, non-threatening way to your child. Most children are scared to start a new school, and our children will show that emotion through anger, temper tantrums, anxiety, or other ways. It is best to take the child at least two to three times to the new school while you accompany them so that they can get used to it. If this isn't an option, take them to the school when no one is there. Walk around and point out where everything is located, such as the lunch room, the music room, and home room. Enlist your child's new teacher by asking him or her to immediately give your child a job when he or she gets into the classroom. This may even be set up beforehand, so it is something your child is looking forward to doing. Any activity relieves our kids' anxiety and keeps them calm.

Wellness centers offer a wide variety of modalities including blood testing, kinesiology, nutrition counseling, aromatherapy, acupuncture, acupressure, hypnotherapy and massage.

CHAPTER 22

Wellness Centers

Most cities have wellness centers that offer various modalities for minimizing ADHD symptoms. We wanted to try other options besides medication, so this seemed like a good idea. The wellness center we chose practiced applied kinesiology, used foot baths for detoxification, and performed something called LZR7 for food sensitivities. We visited the doctor once a week for 12 weeks. I can honestly say that I believe my son was a much better child for the two days after visiting the doctor each week, but in the end there was no long-term improvement. The doctor gave me 10 pages of instructions at the beginning of the treatment that suggested I remove all dyes, preservatives, chocolate, and brown drinks from Alex's diet. There was no information on how to do this or what foods I should feed him. It took me the first 10 weeks while we were on the program to figure out how to eliminate just the dyes without starving my child to death! Most of our kids are picky eaters, and eliminating favorite foods and replacing them with healthier items can be a monumental undertaking.

I could spend time here telling you what I think about LZR7 treatment as well as the other alternative treatments that were offered. Although the letter below is quite long, it summarizes the lack of results and the real frustration I felt at the end of this treatment protocol. This is the actual letter I sent to the doctor at the end of our 12 weeks of treatment. I would like to hear from others that may have undergone this treatment with different results, but below is my final summary.

> Dear Doctor,
>
> I have been reviewing your 12-week treatment program that we just completed with Alex and have some thoughts I would like to share.
>
> I was disappointed by the results of the treatment that Alex received from your wellness center. I know you were disappointed as well. In

retrospect, I am not sure I should have expected a 12-week program to fix a six-year problem. That might have been too optimistic. However, your protocols and treatments may have at least pointed me in the right direction to continue trying to help Alex reduce or remove his behavior issues through diet control.

There are a few concerns I would like to raise. First, you said something in our final evaluation meeting that surprised me. I told you I had put Alex on the Feingold Program diet a week before. You said if I had done that the first week of his treatment, that our outcome would have been dramatically different. I am now totally confused as to what your program was supposed to do. It was my understanding the LZR7 was a treatment that removed sensitivities to foods and other substances. The idea is that everything has a different "footprint" and that LZR7 can eliminate the sensitivities to these footprints. I asked you about half way through the program why I needed to eliminate dyes and preservatives if you could simply eliminate my son's sensitivities to these items. You said that LZR7 would hit these items in the last session we had. That made me wonder why LZR7 didn't handle these substance sensitivities in the first session instead of the last, but I didn't question the approach since I have no experience with LZR7. I wasn't extremely motivated to completely change our family's diet if LZR7 would eliminate the sensitivity to these items; however, I did make some substantial changes in what we ate, especially related to dyes.

When we started LZR7, tests said he was sensitive to seldom-eaten foods like raspberries and tuna fish. At the end, the sensitivities included gluten, casein, potatoes, and brown rice, among others—pretty much everything Alex ate on a daily basis. It seems to me he has taken a step backward if he wasn't sensitive to these foods initially but is today. Maybe there is a plausible explanation for this. I would like to understand LZR7 more completely and know what I should really expect from this therapy. The other problem here is that I don't know what his diet should be. Do I just eliminate dyes and preservatives, or do I also eliminate dairy and gluten? Those are two extremely different diets. How do I even know what to feed him?

If I really was supposed to eliminate dyes, preservatives, brown drinks, and chocolate the first week of the program, I think that was a very unrealistic expectation. In addition, if I was then supposed to put him on the diet proposed for an AB blood type, that became even more confusing. As a wellness doctor, you have lived on a diet free of these substances for years, and it likely seems easy for you and is just part of your lifestyle. Although I think my family's diet is better than most, I would be eliminating at least half the foods in my pantry, and I have very little knowledge as to what to replace them with.

If you ask someone to eliminate half the foods they currently eat, you have to give them some idea how to replace it. I would recommend you add four weeks to the beginning of your program and do a number of nutritional counseling sessions first. If I had a menu going into the week, along with a grocery list, snack list, and recipes, I might be able to learn how to feed my family in a different way. I have spent 30 hours or more in grocery stores over the last 12 weeks reading labels. It is exhausting and frustrating.

Last night my child had a stomachache. I only had a few choices. There was Pepto-Bismol, which had red 27 in it. There were Tums, which had red 40, yellow 6, yellow 7, and blue in it. Or I could just let him hurt. These aren't good options, and if there are others, I need to know what they are! I need a book to read that will tell me what I should do in these situations or at least some helpful hints. I can't believe this is an uncommon problem to have, but I feel like I am the only one in the world who is going through this, and I can't find anyone that will help me.

You have told me what *not to do* but haven't told me what *to do instead*. I am making my way through the maze of online food sources, Trader Joe's, Earth Fare, Fresh Market, and others, and it is a slow, painful process. In the meantime, my son is not getting any better because at least once every three to four days, he eats something that includes a dye or preservative, to which at this point I can only assume he is highly sensitive. Last night I opted for the Pepto-Bismol knowing that it would likely give me three more days of impulsive, confrontational behavior. Probably a bad choice, but it made him feel better, and he finally went to sleep.

I am obviously clueless at this point as to how to best proceed with helping Alex, but I do know that I will not stop until I have the child I know Alex is capable of being.

Sincerely,
Linda Artis

Sorry for making you read the entire letter I sent to this alternative medicine practitioner, but I hope it raises some good points if this is a modality that you are thinking about trying.

After going through the eight-week elimination and detox diet, you will have discovered your child's food sensitivities. You may want to look for a wellness center that offers other modalities to try, such as acupressure or aromatheraphy. Additional food sensitivity testing and detoxification will likely not add much value at this point.

CHAPTER 23

Allergy Testing and Food Sensitivities

I am not a biologist or a chemist. I'm also not a doctor. What I am is a mom with two kids who have a "diagnosis"—a mom who has spent countless hours and dollars helping her children fit into this world.

I don't know all the technical terms for everything I will discuss here, but I believe I can get across the idea. First, I have learned that comparing an allergy to a food intolerance or food sensitivity is like comparing an apple to an orange. They are two entirely different things with different tests and different treatments, so be careful when you talk about these two very different terms to a doctor.

We did food sensitivity testing with Alex, spent a great deal of money and a great deal of time, and were very disappointed in the results. After my personal experiences, I would not recommend food sensitivity testing. If you are interested in your child's food sensitivities, do the elimination diet in part one.

Here is my story on food sensitivity testing. The two tests we did were called the Alcat test and the TRIAD Profile (then by a company called Metametrix and now by Genova Diagnostics). The companies work through licensed doctors' offices. Metametrix sent me a listing of doctors in my area that perform the test. I found a wellness center that had a good reputation. I didn't want to do this testing more than once, so I asked for both tests simultaneously. Although the doctor had never done this, she agreed that in order to test for foods as well as other toxins in the environment that both tests would be helpful.

The Alcat is a blood test. Alex had to go to a clinic and have eight vials of blood drawn. He did an amazing job enduring this procedure. I doubt all kids will do as well as he did. It helped to promise him ice cream immediately after the blood test. Since it was near dinnertime, we agreed to an ice cream sundae for dinner. I think it was such a novelty to him that he sat still and let them take the blood. It was an odd night since we really did eat ice cream for dinner, but it was well worth it.

The same day, we administered the TRIAD Profile, which involves a urine specimen and two finger pricks, one while fasting (first thing in the morning) and one not fasting. As it turned out, that test was much harder than the blood draw. A word of advice—when the package says run your child's hand under hot water for two minutes before doing the prick, do it! Alex refused to do it. We pricked his poor fingers four times, and it was like squeezing blood out of a turnip. Twenty minutes and a lot of screaming later, we were finally done with the first prick. In the afternoon, he decided to follow directions and put his hand under the hot water. One prick and two minutes later, we had all the blood we needed. Then there was more ice cream!

The results arrived three weeks later, and we were called into the doctor's office to review them. I have published the results in figure 1 and figure 2. Each test came back in stark contrast to the other test. Since the doctor had never done both tests at once, she sheepishly admitted that she did not know which one was accurate or if either of them was accurate!

A quick comparison will show that while Alcat said that Alex was severely sensitive to oats, tuna, and strawberries, the TRIAD Profile told me that he had no sensitivity at all to those foods. The TRIAD Profile clearly pointed out that he was severely sensitive to whole eggs, milk, and soybeans, while Alcat assured me that he had no sensitivity at all to those items. As I tried to take items from both tests that caused severe sensitivities out of his diet, it became a disaster not worth pursuing.

Figure 1. **Alcat Food Sensitivity Test**

Negative**	Foods to Avoid		
No Sensitivity	Mild Intolerance	Moderate Intolerance	Severe Intolerance
Almond	Brewers yeast	Basil	Black pepper
Apple	Brussels sprouts	Cabbage	Carob
Barley	Butternut Squash	Chicken	Cottonseed
Beef	Cashew	Cocoa	Green Pea
Broccoli	Cauliflower	Ginger	Oats
Cane sugar	Cherry	Hops	Strawberry
Cantaloupe	Cinnamon	Pecan	Tuna
Carrot	Clam	Rice	
Coconut	Corn	Sesame	
Egg white	Cucumber		
Egg yolk	Eggplant		
Garlic	Lamb		
Green bean	Parsley		
Honey	Peanut		
Lemon	Pear		
Lime	Pinto Bean		
Milk	Plum		
Millet	Pork		
Mustard	Psyllium		
Oregano	Rye		
Peach	Soul		
Pineapple	Yellow squash		
Soybean	Sweet potato		
Tomato	Vanilla		
Turkey	Wheat		

***Partial list of foods*

Figure 2. **TRIAD Profile Bloodspot TM IgG Food Antibodies**

Negative	Foods to Avoid		
No Sensitivity	**Mild +1 and +2**	**Average +3 and +4**	**Severe +5**
Almond	Corn	Mustard seed	Whole egg
Beef	Garlic	Cashews	Milk
Cantaloupe	Pinto beans		Peanut
Chicken			Soybean
Crab			
Lobster			
Oats			
Orange			
Green peas			
Pork			
Rice			
Salmon			
Shrimp			
Strawberry			
Sunflower			
Tomato			
Tuna			
Turkey			
Walnut			
Wheat			

Instead of going to a great deal of expense and effort on these tests, spend some time reading part one and conduct your own elimination diet. This a good way to determine your child's food sensitivities and is a much less expensive approach.

In general, I believe food sensitivities are almost always part of ADHD but are seldom 100 percent of the problem. Other moms have told me this as well. Removing the majority of your child's ADHD symptoms takes a building-block approach, and starting with food sensitivities is the foundation.

CHAPTER 24

Medication

I don't believe that medication is ever the permanent fix for our children's diagnoses, but there is a place for medication. When I first realized what a significant struggle my daughter was having in school, a friend of mine suggested I put her on a drug called Focalin. I never wanted to medicate my children, but the justification went something like this: You know your child is struggling and is becoming increasingly unhappy. You could try a stimulant drug and see what happens. If it helps her to focus, makes her happier, and increases her satisfaction with school, then why wouldn't you keep her on the drug? You can always take her off the drug, but if you don't try it, you will never know if it will help her enough to justify taking it.

It is then your choice as a parent to continue looking for a better solution or to continue medicating your child into adulthood. Some children do outgrow their ADHD or learn skills to live with the symptoms. There isn't a right or wrong answer to this dilemma. Everyone's answer will be different, just as every child will heal differently and parents will do their best with the circumstances they were dealt.

There are entire books written on ADHD medications. If you are interested in pursuing this route, contact your pediatrician. He or she probably will administer a basic ADHD test and then prescribe the drug of choice. If your child is already taking medication, you can still go through both eight-week programs in this book. Once you notice your child calming down after the elimination diet, you may choose to work with your pediatrician to decrease the dosage or eliminate medication completely.

A pediatrician will typically prescribe medication, a naturopathic or homeopathic doctor will create a treatment plan to remove foods and toxins based on testing and questionaires, and a physchologist, phychiatrist or a therapist will work with your child to help with social skills. Each has it's own merits.

CHAPTER 25

Psychiatric Professionals

When we were going through the *Celebrate Calm* program, we needed to seek out a psychiatric professional for help. Alex was so obstinate that he wouldn't talk to the counselor. She would ask questions, and he would answer with a yes or no or totally ignore her if it was an open-ended question. After six months of this behavior, we gave up on this intervention.

That is our story, but I have talked to families who have found excellent counselors who have helped their children through anxious times. If you can find someone who can help your child, and you can afford the fees or insurance will pay for the sessions, it is probably worth giving this a try. It won't heal the ADHD, but it can help a child through anxiety in different situations.

Many of our children suffer from lack of social skills, especially with a diagnosis such as Asperger's. A good counselor or group session can help teach our kids age-appropriate social skills.

In just a few short years,
Brain Balance has expanded
its operations in the
United States to over 100 branches.

CHAPTER 26

Brain Balance

I don't have any personal experience with Brain Balance, other than taking my son in for the initial assessment test and calling a few references. The Brain Balance website states: "The Brain Balance Program® is the most comprehensive approach to overcoming the symptoms of ADHD, learning disabilities, processing disorders, Asperger's syndrome, and a host of other related childhood learning and developmental issues. Our cutting-edge, integrated approach combines three core modalities into one."

The first modality is Academic Activities. The idea is that certain areas of our children's brains are underdeveloped. Because certain academic subjects are more difficult, our kids stay away from them and focus on the areas in which they excel. This continues to worsen the imbalance unless a program such as Brain Balance is utilized to concentrate on the less-developed parts of their brains and to strengthen those areas with focused attention.

The second modality is Sensory Motor Activities. The brain is built first on movement and sensory stimulation, so Brain Balance activities first focus on this key part of brain development. The Brain Balance website states, "Improving motor skills, sensory detection, and processing has to come before any higher learning, either behaviorally or academically, can take place." This is accomplished through a number of different physical activities that focus on muscle tone, rhythm, gross and fine-motor skills, primitive and postural reflexes, and other physical attributes.

The third modality is called the Balance 360 Clean-Eating Nutrition System. This is a step-by-step approach to a balanced diet.

Brain Balance offers various short seminars on a regular basis in order to expose interested parents to some of the methods they use to help treat symptoms. An assessment is required first and then you will sign up for three sessions per week at the Brain Balance facility for the first three months, as well as doing daily exercises. After the three months there is a re-assessment process.

I have no knowledge of how successful Brain Balance is or is not. I only know when I was considering it, I felt it would have been difficult to get my very defiant child to the facility three days a week and also perform the exercises at home on the other days of the week.

Other Alternatives

I have listed only a handful of the most common ADHD interventions. Plenty of other, less mainstream approaches to diminish or eliminate symptoms are out there. I don't have any first-hand experience with other approaches; however, I am open to the idea that lots of other options exist and might be helpful.

Please check out my website (LindaArtis.com) and comment on other alternative treatments that you might have found useful. I am a firm believer that moms can help other moms to end our kids' and our families' suffering.

Epilogue

As I was going through various interventions with Alex, I always thought that I should write a book. I was learning so much about how to cope with different diagnoses, but I didn't think I should write a book if I didn't have a happy ending. My friends would keep pushing me to write, and I would keep saying that I couldn't write anything until I knew how it was going to end. I intermittently wrote some pages as I went through various interventions, but I was ultimately waiting for that silver bullet that would heal Alex completely and give me a great ending to my story.

That didn't happen. In retrospect, I was naïve to think that any one intervention would cure Alex. If that were the case, then someone else would have figured it all out by now. That being said, there are children who find extreme relief from ADHD and ODD symptoms with just one intervention, which is typically food sensitivities. Many require a building-block approach.

I have written extensively about Alex and a little about Heather and their struggles in life. I have told you about Alex's terrible behavior and Heather's school struggles with her inability to focus. As I have been through different interventions, I believe some have been helpful and some have not been, but the ones that have been helpful have built on each other. I don't believe any one intervention would have worked for either of my children.

Alex is finishing up sixth grade as I write this epilogue and has grown into a funny, intelligent, self-confident child. Somewhere along the way, his anger melted into something less dangerous. He still has an occasional outburst and can still be stubborn, but his entire demeanor has changed. I received an email from his middle school youth director at church not too long ago. Alex wanted to help out with a babysitting project, and the exchange went like this:

> **Youth Director:** "Please have your children at the church at noon and remind them that this is a time for them to babysit younger children, not a time for them to play. Thank you!"
>
> **Me:** "Got it! I know Alex can be a real handful sometimes (actually most of the time). Please feel free to touch base with me at any time if you need help with discipline issues."
>
> **Youth Director:** "Honestly, you prepared me, but I have yet to have one issue to date. He is always respectful and under control. Truly!"

I cried when I received that response. Every time I go back and read that email, I cry. I never thought I would read an email like this about my son. A few years ago I couldn't imagine anyone saying anything like this about my child. These days, much of my anger and frustration are morphing into pride and joy as I watch my child grow into the person he wants to be. He makes me laugh, and even when he gets into trouble at school, usually for doing something I think is more funny than bad, we work through it together. I don't get mad and yell anymore. He is a smart child and often thinks outside the box. Sometimes he is going to try to play the system just because he can. That isn't necessarily a bad thing as long as it doesn't go too far and isn't morally wrong. If it does get out of hand, Alex and I both know that I will be there for him. I will be there not only to bail him out but also to offer suggestions on how it should be done the next time. I trust that he is capable of handling the same situation better in the future. If he doesn't fail sometimes, he will never learn how to live a healthy productive life.

My strongest desire is for each of you reading this to feel the pride and joy that should be a part of every parent's life. Being on high alert every minute you are with your child is exhausting. This is hard work, but it can be done. I hope I have inspired you to try some new interventions that you may not have considered or some that you knew about but didn't know how to go about implementing.

Good luck and God bless!

Glossary

ADD: attention deficit disorder is no longer a widely used term. Although it is very confusing, the medical profession now prefers to label ADD as "ADHD without hyperactivity."

ADHD: attention deficit hyperactivity disorder is a chronic condition that affects millions of children and often continues into adulthood. ADHD includes a combination of persistent problems, such as difficulty sustaining attention, hyperactivity, and impulsive behavior.

Asperger syndrome: one of several previously separate subtypes of autism that were folded into the single diagnosis, autism spectrum disorder (ASD) with the publication of the DSM-5 diagnostic manual in 2013. Asperger syndrome was generally considered to be on the "high functioning" end of the spectrum. Affected children and adults have difficulty with social interactions and exhibit a restricted range of interests and/or repetitive behaviors. Motor development may be delayed, leading to clumsiness or uncoordinated motor movements.

BHA & BHT: butylated hydroxyanisole (BHA) and butylated hydroxytoluene (BHT) are widely used by the food industry as preservatives, mainly to prevent oils in foods from oxidizing and becoming rancid. Based on animal studies, the National Toxicology Program has concluded that BHA "is reasonably anticipated to be a human carcinogen."

food allergy: an immune system response that typically occurs almost immediately after even the tiniest amount of a food is consumed. Symptoms can include digestive problems, hives, or swollen airways.

food sensitivity or food intolerance: a digestive system response to a particular food that is ingested. Symptoms can include intestinal gas, abdominal pain, diarrhea, headache, or sluggishness.

ODD: oppositional defiant disorder is a childhood disorder characterized by negative, defiant, disobedient, and often hostile behavior primarily focused toward adults and authority figures.

RAD: reactive attachment disorder is caused by a lack of attachment to any specific caregiver at an early age and results in an inability for the child to form normal, loving relationships with others.

TBHQ: tertiary butylhydroquinone is commonly used in foods such as crackers, microwave popcorn, butter, and chicken nuggets to preserve freshness.

About the Author

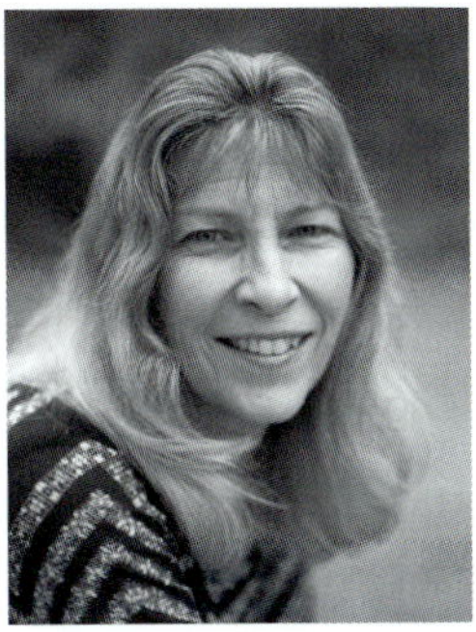

Linda Artis has two children who have been diagnosed with ADD, ADHD, and RAD. She has spent the past 12 years working through various interventions to heal her children and help them to live more peaceful, fulfilling lives. This has included working with dozens of different interventions, from medications and counseling to food sensitivities and toxin removal. This book, *Healing Our ADHD Children*, is a summary of hundreds of hours of research and personal triumphs of children who have greatly diminished their symptoms without the use of medication.

Linda Artis owned, operated, and helped grow a multi-million dollar accounting firm for 23 years. She retired at the age of 50. As she became more in touch with her spirituality, her higher purpose in life began to emerge. She became an author and is passionate about helping others navigate the pitfalls of childhood diagnoses such as ADHD. She lives in Charlotte, North Carolina.